Respiratory Medicine

Respiratory Medicine offers clinical and research-oriented resources for pulmonologists and other practitioners and researchers interested in respiratory care. Spanning a broad range of clinical and research issues in respiratory medicine, the series covers such topics as COPD, asthma and allergy, pulmonary problems in pregnancy, molecular basis of lung disease, sleep disordered breathing, and others.

The series editors are Sharon Rounds, MD, Professor of Medicine and of Pathology and Laboratory Medicine at the Alpert Medical School at Brown University, Anne Dixon, MD, Professor of Medicine and Director of the Division of Pulmonary and Critical Care at Robert Larner, MD College of Medicine at the University of Vermont, and Lynn M. Schnapp, MD, George R. And Elaine Love Professor and Chair of Medicine at the University of Wisconsin-Madison School of Medicine and Public Health.

Erik R. Swenson • Andrew M. Luks
Editors

The Lungs at the Extremes of Environment and Age

Springer

Editors
Erik R. Swenson
Department of Medicine
Dartmouth Hitchcock Medical Center
Lebanon, NH, USA

Andrew M. Luks
Department of Medicine
University of Washington
Seattle, WA, USA

ISSN 2197-7372 ISSN 2197-7380 (electronic)
Respiratory Medicine
ISBN 978-3-031-98370-2 ISBN 978-3-031-98371-9 (eBook)
https://doi.org/10.1007/978-3-031-98371-9

This Springer imprint is published by the registered company Springer Nature Switzerland AG
The registered company address is: Gewerbestrasse 11, 6330 Cham, Switzerland

Preface

Of all the organs in humans, the lungs by virtue of their vast surface area necessary for efficient gas exchange are most unique in the extent to which they are exposed to the external environment and sensitive to a variety of stresses, including changes in barometric pressure, as can occur with travel to high altitude or underwater or with changes in temperature, humidity, metabolic demands, and other factors. We evolved in the temperate terrestrial lowlands of continental Africa, but in migrating "out of Africa" humans now either live permanently in challenging environments or are frequently exposed to them on a temporary basis with work, recreation, or exploration, which poses special challenges to the lungs' function and integrity that were not anticipated or selected for in our early evolution. This book entitled *The Lungs at the Extremes of Enviornment and Age* explores the aspects of lung physiology and anatomy across the spectrum of age as well as a broad range of extreme environments that demonstrate both the resilience of the lungs and the dangers and consequences of pushing the frontiers of our existence.

The first chapter focuses on the ranges of temperature and humidity that the lungs experience in various environments and their ability to condition inspired air to protect the delicate alveolar–capillary barrier and to contribute to heat dissipation. The second chapter explores the unique challenges of diving, both breathing compressed gases for extended underwater periods and depths and breath-hold diving at extreme depths. The third chapter discusses the challenges posed at high altitude with a focus on the ventilatory responses required to deal with the lower oxygen content of inspired air and the stress on the pulmonary circulation. The fourth chapter explores short- and long-term impact on the lungs of the newest of mankind's migration, that of the weightlessness of space travel. The subject of the fifth chapter is exercise and the challenges the lungs face in maintaining effective gas exchange in the face of greater than 20-fold increases in metabolic demand from that at rest. The sixth chapter on the comparative physiology of lungs and other gas exchanging organs in the vertebrate phylum offers interesting comparisons and differences in their respiratory organs and how other creatures handle their challenging environments. The last two chapters focus on lung function at the extremes of age, including the challenge of transitioning to air breathing in the formerly liquid filled lungs at the time of birth and changes in lung function toward the end of life. We are grateful to all the authors who have contributed their expertise in their areas and hope that their contributions will renew our awe of the lungs and how they have been able to take us far beyond our earliest existence as a species.

Lebanon, NH, USA Erik R. Swenson
Seattle, WA, USA Andrew M. Luks

Contents

The original version of the book has been revised. A correction to these chapters can be found at https://doi.org/10.1007/978-3-031-98371-9_9

Contributors

Marc Moritz Berger Department of Anesthesiology, Intensive Care Medicine, Emergency Medicine and Pain Therapy, RKH Hospital Ludwigsburg, Ludwigsburg, Germany

Wiaam Elkhatib MD MPH, Division of Public Health, Infectious Disease and Occupational Medicine; Aerospace Medicine, Mayo Clinic, Rochester, MN, USA

Catherine M. Ivy Department of Biology, University of Saskatchewan, Saskatoon, SK, Canada

David A. Kaminsky Pulmonary and Critical Care, University of Vermont Larner College of Medicine, Burlington, VT, USA

Deborah R. Liptzin Department of Pediatrics, University of Washington, Seattle, WA, USA

Harold L. Manning Dartmouth-Hitchcock Medical Center, Geisel School of Medicine at Dartmouth, Hanover, NH, USA

Dakota McNierney DO, Division of Pulmonary and Sleep Medicine, Department of Medicine, Mayo Clinic, Phoenix, AZ, USA
Department of Critical Care Medicine, Mayo Clinic, Phoenix, AZ, USA

Weston T. Powell Department of Pediatrics, University of Washington, Seattle, WA, USA

Jan Stepanek MD MPH, Aerospace Medicine Program, Department of Medicine, Mayo Clinic, Phoenix, AZ, USA

Kay Tetzlaff Department of Sports Medicine, University Hospital Tübingen, Tübingen, Germany

Andrew Tomlinson University of Texas Southwestern Medical Center, Dallas, TX, USA

Chapter 1
Breathing at Extremes of Temperature and Humidity

David A. Kaminsky

Introduction

The lungs are a unique organ because they are in direct contact with the external environment. As such, they must deal with extremes of environmental conditions, in particular, temperature and humidity. A primary purpose of the upper airway is to condition inspired air so that it reaches body conditions of temperature and humidity (37 °C and 100% saturated) in the alveolar space. Since ambient air is typically much cooler and drier than alveolar air, the lungs must give up heat and humidity to the air to achieve this conditioning. If left unchecked, the body would ultimately cool down and dry out if there were no way to replenish heat and humidity lost to the air. Fortunately, we are designed to breathe in a bidirectional fashion such that heat and humidity given up on inspiration can be recovered, at least to some degree, during expiration. In addition to conditioning the inspired air, the lungs must deal with the consequences of alterations in temperature and humidity of the air on breathing and health in general. This chapter will explore the mechanisms of air conditioning by the lungs and how varying temperature and humidity affect lung function. In particular, this chapter will highlight exercise-induced bronchospasm, implications for patients on mechanical ventilation or with a laryngectomy, and the effects of changes in environmental temperature and humidity on breathing in people with or without chronic lung disease.

D. A. Kaminsky (✉)
Pulmonary and Critical Care, University of Vermont Larner College of Medicine, Burlington, VT, USA
e-mail: David.kaminsky@uvm.edu

E. R. Swenson, A. M. Luks (eds.), *The Lungs at the Extremes of Environment and Age*, Respiratory Medicine, https://doi.org/10.1007/978-3-031-98371-9_1

The Lung as a Thermodynamic Regulator of Inspired Air Conditions

Air entering the respiratory tract must be warmed and humidified to body conditions to minimize the irritating and potentially damaging effects of cold and dryness on the respiratory mucosa [1]. Conditioning of inspired air starts with the nose. The extensive turbinate structure of the nose allows for a relatively large surface area to promote an exchange of heat and water to warm and humidify inspired air [2] (Fig. 1.1). Heat is extracted from the airway walls, and water is evaporated from the airway surface liquid to warm and humidify the incoming air. The respiratory epithelium is cooled and dried from this loss of heat and water, so that on expiration, heat and water transfer back again as expired air passes over the epithelium. This results in the temperature of the exhaled air being reduced relative to air in the alveolar space [3, 4]. Complex mathematical modeling reveals the lung to be well-engineered to fully condition the inhaled air, even under conditions of high minute ventilation, and to be relatively efficient at returning up to 50% of the extracted heat and water to the airway during exhalation [5]. Interestingly, across mammals, the efficiency of air conditioning in the nose is proportional not only to the mass of the animal but their maximal running speed, suggesting that proper conditioning of inspired air is critical to physical performance [1]. At rest, the point at which inspired air becomes fully saturated and body temperature—isothermal saturation boundary (ISB)—is estimated to be about 5 cm below the carina, but it may penetrate deeper when breathing cold, dry air or breathing at elevated minute ventilation [6]. During hyperpnea, as occurs with exercise, nose breathing shifts to combined nose-and-mouth breathing when ventilation exceeds ~30 l/min, thus setting up a situation where air can no longer be adequately conditioned by the nose. McFadden and colleagues showed that the heating and humidification of ambient air involved the intrathoracic airways beyond the extrathoracic airways (nose/oropharynx), and this

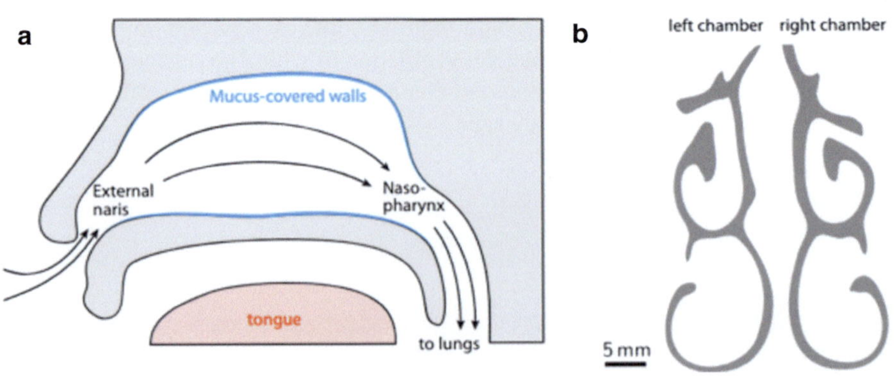

Fig. 1.1 Nasal airflow and anatomy. As inspired air flows through the nose (**a**), the cross-sectional shape of the nasal turbinates (**b**) provides a relatively large surface area for effective warming and humidification. (Modified from [56] with permission from PNAS)

effect penetrated deeper into the airways as the level of ventilation increased [7, 8] (Fig. 1.2).

Besides hyperpnea, another circumstance that affects the position of the ISB is mechanical ventilation through an endotracheal tube. In this case, the upper airway is bypassed, so warming and humidifying the air must take place lower in the respiratory tract. Consequently, the ISB is shifted deeper into the lung [6]. Excessive cooling and drying of the lower airways can result in damage to the respiratory epithelium with cough, bronchospasm, thick secretions, mucus plugging, airway obstruction, infection, and increased work of breathing. Therefore, it is essential that the inspired air used during mechanical ventilation be warmed and humidified prior to entering the lungs. Different external heated humidifiers, or heat and moisture exchangers (HMEs), can be used, but neither holds a distinct advantage over

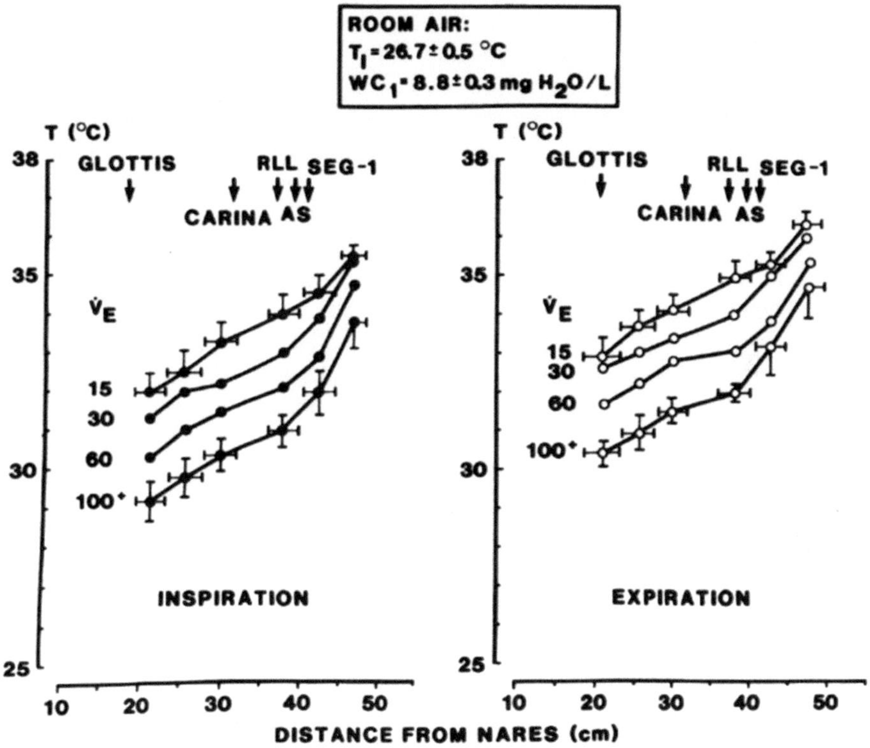

Fig. 1.2 Thermal mapping of the airways in healthy volunteers. Temperature (*y*-axis) is shown relative to the distance of the measurement from the nares (*x*-axis). Air is warmer on both inspiration and expiration as the measurement is taken deeper within the bronchial tree, and is warmer on expiration than inspiration for any given distance. Air temperature is also modified by the level of hyperpnea shown by the different relationships of temperature vs. distance based on minute ventilation ($\dot{V}_E$). Higher $\dot{V}_E$ results in cooler starting temperatures and slightly lower warmer final temperatures as measurement proceeds from 20 to 50 cm from the nares. (Reproduced from [8] with permission from the American Physiological Society)

the other [9]. It is equally important to use humidified gas during non-invasive ventilation or in patients on continuous positive airway pressure (CPAP) therapy to prevent nasal/oral dryness [10] or in patients with a laryngectomy (via an HME) [11]. Providing warmed and humidified air is also an essential component that allows the delivery of high-flow nasal cannula oxygen [12].

The Effects of Extremes of Ambient Temperature and Humidity on Lung Function

Exposure to cold air can cause airflow obstruction even at rest or when just the face or nose is exposed to cold air [13–15]. Whole-body exposure to cold can also result in exercise-induced bronchospasm (EIB) among people with asthma [16]. Repeated exposure to cold air among non-asthmatic athletes can result in up to 75% having airway hyperresponsiveness to methacholine, implicating cold air airway injury as a possible cause of airway hyperresponsiveness [17]. While increased inflammatory cells have been found in the airways of athletes exposed to cold air, it is not clear whether these represent chronic or adaptive changes [18]. One study has found an increased prevalence of newly diagnosed asthma in the 1–2 years following a cold winter with below-normal average temperatures [19]. While this finding suggests that prolonged exposure to cold temperatures may lead to the development of asthma, the authors acknowledge that other unmeasured related exposures, such as indoor air pollutants, may also be involved.

Exposure to extreme heat may occur as a result of combustion. Thermal injury is typically limited to the upper airway and results in erythema, edema, ulceration, and excessive secretions [20]. Such an injury may be life-threatening. Intubation may be required, but deciding who and when to intubate remains a complex clinical decision given that, in some cases, prophylactic intubation may be unnecessary [21].

The effects of humidity on lung function are complex. While low heat/humidity appears to exacerbate EIB, many patients with asthma say humidity worsens their symptoms [22]. Since house dust mites and mold are both known to be more prevalent in humid conditions, it has been postulated that the association of worsened asthma symptoms with humidity may be due to the effects of these two common environmental allergens in patients with asthma rather than the humidity, per se [23, 24]. One study attempted to sort out the association of allergic sensitization to dust mites and mold and the effect of humidity on asthma symptoms but found that the association with humidity was an independent effect [25]. At rest, humidity has little effect on lung function [26]. However, during exercise, high humidity has been demonstrated to cause a transient fall in airway conductance, postulated to be due to deposition of excess water on the airway epithelium rendering it hypo-osmolar and thus causing an irritant response [27]. In addition, 100% relative humidity has been shown to destabilize surfactant films [28], perhaps contributing to airway closure during exercise under high humidity.

The Effects of Temperature and Humidity in the Work Environment

Low and high temperatures in the work environment can have adverse effects on health and work performance. A recent review suggested that the optimal temperature is 22–24 °C for temperate or cold climates to prevent respiratory symptoms and inflammation and optimize work performance [29]. Similarly, relative humidities of 40–60% are best to prevent dry larynx, nose, eyes, and airways on the one hand (<40%), and excessive overgrowth and exposure to dust mites and molds on the other hand (>60%).

The Effects of Acutely Cooling and Drying the Airways on Lung Function

A common manifestation of asthma is exercise-induced bronchospasm (EIB). It has long been recognized that certain activities and environments appear to be associated more commonly with EIB than others. These activities involve exercise that results in high levels of sustained ventilation, such as running, swimming, rowing, and skiing, and environments that are cool and dry, such as winter sports or indoor hockey arenas. Based on these observations, there is debate in the literature about whether cooling or drying of the airways is the primary stimulus for EIB [30]. Since the laws of thermodynamics mandate that cooling occurs at a surface where evaporation takes place (conservation of energy), both stimuli are necessarily present. The classic presentation involves an athlete who develops symptoms of EIB (cough, wheezing, chest tightness, shortness of breath) within minutes of stopping their activity, but typically not during the activity itself [31]. The diagnosis can be confirmed by formal testing with exercise or hyperpnea challenge that results in a 10–15% fall in FEV_1 from baseline, which typically occurs during the first 5–15 min following the challenge (Fig. 1.3). The EIB response varies depending on the relative conditions of the exercise environment versus the recovery environment [32]. For example, EIB is less severe when exercising and recovering in a warm, humid environment, but is typically more severe when exercise takes place in a cool environment and recovery occurs in a warm, humid one. This leads to two competing theories accounting for airway narrowing. One view is that cooling is the initial stimulus, which then leads to rapid rewarming by excessive reactive hyperemia and, consequently, edema of the airway wall in an effort to restore heat and humidity to the airway epithelium [33, 34]. The other is that drying of the airway is the initial stimulus, which then leads to an increase in local osmolality of the airway lining fluid [35], resulting in stimulation of airway epithelial cells, mast cells, and eosinophils to release bronchoconstricting agents like histamine and leukotrienes. While there are compelling data supporting both hypotheses, clever experiments have demonstrated that the drying of the airway appears to be the key stimulus [36–38].

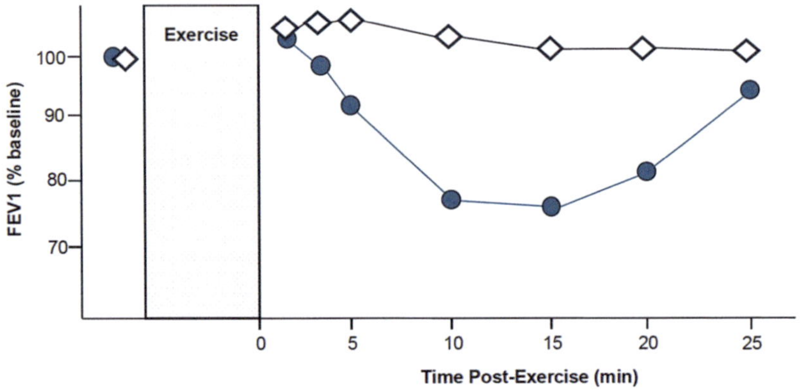

Fig. 1.3 Depiction of classic response demonstrating exercise-induced bronchospasm. Following baseline measurement of FEV_1, the patient exercises to achieve a high level of minute ventilation for 6 min (hashed box), following which FEV_1 measurements are repeated over a short recovery time. While the healthy person (diamonds) may demonstrate a transient increase in FEV_1 following exercise, the person with EIB (circles) has a fall in FEV1 that exceeds 10–15% from baseline in the first few minutes following exercise, and then slowly recovers spontaneously by 30–45 min after the challenge

Activation of resident airway epithelial cells, mast cells, and eosinophils may then lead to airway inflammation [39, 40]. In addition, there is evidence that surfactant function might also be reduced, which would be expected to lead to enhanced airway closure [40]. Since the downstream effect of cooling and drying the airway is bronchoconstriction and inflammation, bronchodilators together with inhaled steroids or anti-leukotriene agents are the mainstays of treatment of EIB [31]. Heat and moisture-exchanging breathing devices (HMEs) have been shown to mitigate EIB, but they also increase airflow resistance and, as a result, may affect athletic performance [41].

Effect of Climate Change-Induced Alterations of Temperature and Humidity

Climate change is a major public health issue among patients with respiratory disease [42]. Besides extremes of temperature, multiple other effects of climate change are implicated in causing adverse health effects, including droughts, wildfires, and rainstorms with flooding and subsequent increases in mold and other aeroallergens. In addition, changes in temperature and humidity may enhance the adverse respiratory health effects of air pollution, including ozone, oxides of nitrogen, and particulates [43]. For example, in a study of 1103 elderly men from 1995 to 2011, an increase in temperature and an increase in relative humidity were both associated with small decreases in lung function as measured by spirometry [44]. These associations were strongest within the first 2 days of temperature change and the first 6 days of humidity change. Interestingly, the associations were stronger when combined with higher exposures to black carbon as an indicator of air pollution. Air pollution also modified the effect of changes in relative humidity in a cohort of adolescents from Germany, where an increase in relative humidity was associated with a significant decrease in FEV_1 on high ozone days [45]. Similar findings were shown among people 40–80 years old in China, where cadmium, nickel, ozone, and ultrafine particle pollution were particularly important [43].

Among the offspring of participants of the Framingham Heart Study, higher outdoor air temperatures were associated with lower FEV_1 and FVC, but this was seen only in winter and spring [46]. Similarly, increased outdoor air pollution as assessed by particulate matter <2.5 µm (PM2.5) was associated with lower lung function, but only on unseasonably warm but not unseasonably cool days (Fig. 1.4). These observations led the authors to speculate that behavioral changes may explain the findings because people may be more likely to engage in outdoor physical activities when the weather warms up outside.

The effects of climate change on temperature and humidity may also exacerbate underlying chronic respiratory disease. A general survey of patients with chronic obstructive pulmonary disease (COPD) in Canada revealed that both hot/humid and cold/dry environmental conditions were associated with reduced physical activity and worse health status, with hot/humid conditions associated with exacerbations of

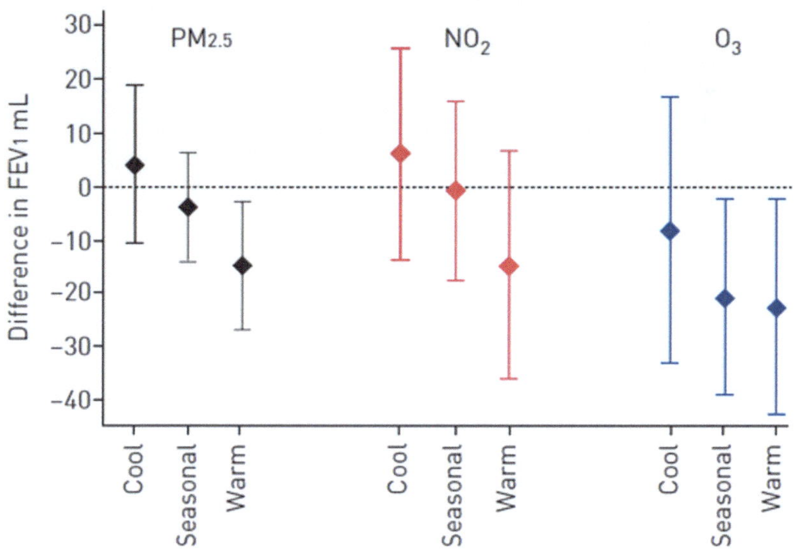

Fig. 1.4 Relationship of change in FEV_1 to ambient particulate matter <2.5-µm diameter (PM2.5), nitrogen dioxide (NO_2), or ozone (O_3) in the air during different relative temperatures. Compared to when temperatures are seasonal or cooler for that time of year, warmer temperatures are associated with greater falls in FEV_1. (Reproduced from [46] with permission from the European Respiratory Society)

COPD [47]. Extremes of temperature are associated with worsening symptoms of asthma, with cold conditions affecting hospital visits more than hot conditions [48]. Various mechanisms have been implicated beyond the cooling and drying of the mucosa, resulting in bronchoconstriction as in EIB. These include increased inflammation from exposures to both extremes of temperature [49], fluxes in temperature or humidity that result in increased viral activity (e.g., influenza) that could trigger asthma flares [50], increased temperature-induced injury resulting in the production of heat shock protein (HSP)-mediated inflammation [51], and activation of temperature-sensitive transient receptor potential (TRP) ion channels that can result in neurogenic inflammation [52]. Climate change effects will not only lead to the potential for more symptoms from asthma, COPD, and other chronic lung disease but also to increased pulmonary infections [53].

Hospital admissions for respiratory and cardiovascular diseases are also associated with ambient temperature and humidity. In the study by Lin and colleagues, hospital admission rates between 1991 and 2004 increased above a threshold of 29.4 °C and were worse when relative humidity was high [54] (Fig. 1.5). Among Medicare beneficiaries across 120 cities, the high temperature was associated with increased hospitalization for all-cause respiratory disease, mainly infections and

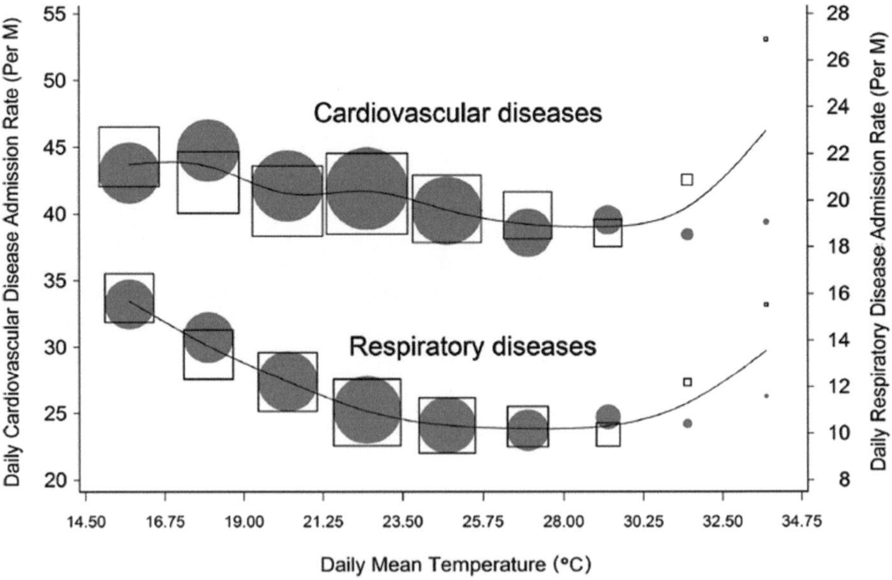

Fig. 1.5 Daily admission rates for cardiovascular disease (left *y*-axis) and respiratory disease (right *y*-axis) based on daily mean temperature and humidity. Circles represent daily mean admission rates when humidity was below the median, and squares represent daily mean admission rates when humidity was above the median, plotted at specific temperatures. The size of the circles and squares is proportional to the number of cases at each temperature range. Notice that there is little interaction of temperature and humidity except at higher temperatures, where high humidity (i.e., hot and humid) is associated with higher hospitalization rates. (Reproduced from [54] with permission from Wolters Kluwer Health, Inc.)

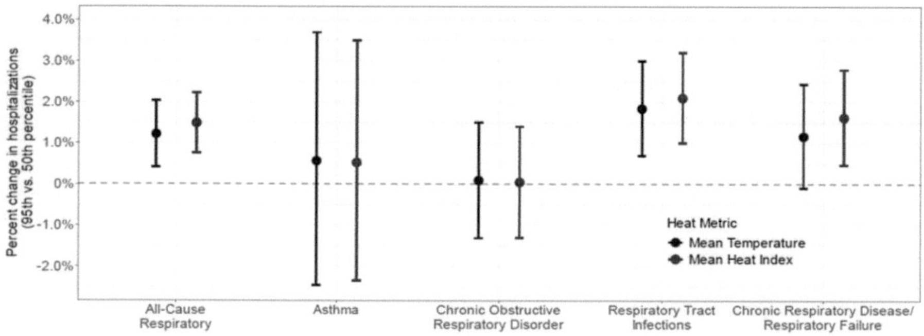

Fig. 1.6 Change in hospitalizations relative to disease state based on mean temperature and heat index. Notice that rates are slightly higher for heat index than temperature for all-cause respiratory, respiratory tract infections, and chronic respiratory disease/respiratory failure, indicating that high humidity has an added detrimental effect to temperature alone. (Reproduced from [55] with permission from American Thoracic Society)

respiratory failure [55]. The association was stronger when using the heat index, which takes into account humidity as well as temperature (Fig. 1.6). There was considerable variation in the association across regions, and it was especially higher among elderly and Black individuals, suggesting socioeconomic and other local environmental factors were involved beyond just temperature and humidity. Interestingly, the risk of temperature and humidity-associated respiratory disease exacerbation was lowest in the Southeast and Southwest, which the authors speculated might be due to higher use of air conditioning and better adaptation of people to heat in these regions. It is important to point out, however, that repeated exposure to indoor cool air as found in air-conditioned environments may carry its own risk in terms of detrimental effects on indoor air quality and promotion of respiratory infections [41].

Conclusions

Extremes of temperature and humidity affect lung function and respiratory health in many ways. Acute exposures to cold, dry air, particularly during the hyperpnea of exercise, result in airway drying and cooling that can penetrate well into the lung periphery and result in airway injury and inflammation manifesting as EIB. Bypassing the normal warming and humidifying function of the nose and upper airway, as in patients on mechanical ventilation or with laryngectomies, can result in respiratory symptoms from excessive drying of secretions, mucus plugging, and airway irritation and inflammation. Chronic exposures to extremes of temperature and humidity occur in everyday life but may become more common during climate change, and these may also result in decrements in lung function and exacerbations of respiratory symptoms, particularly associated with asthma and COPD. Clinicians need to be aware of these important aspects of the environment that can have such a significant impact on the respiratory health of patients and take steps to mitigate these effects. Clinicians also need to educate their patients so they can avoid extremes of temperature and humidity whenever possible.

References

1. Rigaut C, Giaprakis A, Deruyver L, Goole J, Lambert P, Haut B. The air conditioning in the nose of mammals depends on their mass and on their maximal running speed. Sci Rep. 2024;14(1):9053.
2. Elad D, Wolf M, Keck T. Air-conditioning in the human nasal cavity. Respir Physiol Neurobiol. 2008;163(1–3):121–7.
3. Haut B, Nonclercq A, Buess A, Rabineau J, Rigaut C, Sobac B. Comprehensive analysis of heat and water exchanges in the human lungs. Front Physiol. 2021;12:649497.
4. McFadden ER Jr. Heat and water exchange in human airways. Am Rev Respir Dis. 1992;146(5 Pt 2):S8–10.
5. Haut B, Karamaoun C, Mauroy B, Sobac B. Water and heat exchanges in mammalian lungs. Sci Rep. 2023;13(1):6636.
6. Al Ashry HS, Modrykamien AM. Humidification during mechanical ventilation in the adult patient. Biomed Res Int. 2014;2014:715434.
7. McFadden ER Jr, Denison DM, Waller JF, Assoufi B, Peacock A, Sopwith T. Direct recordings of the temperatures in the tracheobronchial tree in normal man. J Clin Invest. 1982;69(3):700–5.
8. McFadden ER Jr, Pichurko BM, Bowman HF, Ingenito E, Burns S, Dowling N, et al. Thermal mapping of the airways in humans. J Appl Physiol (1985). 1985;58(2):564–70.
9. Gillies D, Todd DA, Foster JP, Batuwitage BT. Heat and moisture exchangers versus heated humidifiers for mechanically ventilated adults and children. Cochrane Database Syst Rev. 2017;9(9):Cd004711.
10. Esquinas Rodriguez AM, Scala R, Soroksky A, BaHammam A, de Klerk A, Valipour A, et al. Clinical review: humidifiers during non-invasive ventilation—key topics and practical implications. Crit Care. 2012;16(1):203.
11. Zuur JK, Muller SH, de Jongh FH, van Zandwijk N, Hilgers FJ. The physiological rationale of heat and moisture exchangers in post-laryngectomy pulmonary rehabilitation: a review. Eur Arch Otorrinolaringol. 2006;263(1):1–8.
12. Nishimura M. High-flow nasal cannula oxygen therapy in adults: physiological benefits, indication, clinical benefits, and adverse effects. Respir Care. 2016;61(4):529–41.
13. Berk JL, Lenner KA, McFadden ER Jr. Cold-induced bronchoconstriction: role of cutaneous reflexes vs. direct airway effects. J Appl Physiol (1985). 1987;63(2):659–64.
14. Koskela H, Tukiainen H. Facial cooling, but not nasal breathing of cold air, induces bronchoconstriction: a study in asthmatic and healthy subjects. Eur Respir J. 1995;8(12):2088–93.
15. Koskela HO. Cold air-provoked respiratory symptoms: the mechanisms and management. Int J Circumpolar Health. 2007;66(2):91–100.
16. Koskela H, Tukiainen H, Kononoff A, Pekkarinen H. Effect of whole-body exposure to cold and wind on lung function in asthmatic patients. Chest. 1994;105(6):1728–31.
17. Karjalainen EM, Laitinen A, Sue-Chu M, Altraja A, Bjermer L, Laitinen LA. Evidence of airway inflammation and remodeling in ski athletes with and without bronchial hyperresponsiveness to methacholine. Am J Respir Crit Care Med. 2000;161(6):2086–91.
18. Bonsignore MR, Morici G, Vignola AM, Riccobono L, Bonanno A, Profita M, et al. Increased airway inflammatory cells in endurance athletes: what do they mean? Clin Exp Allergy. 2003;33(1):14–21.

19. Belachew AB, Rantala AK, Jaakkola MS, Hugg TT, Ruuhela R, Kukkonen J, et al. Effect of cold winters on the risk of new asthma: a case-crossover study in Finland. Occup Environ Med. 2023;80(12):702–5.
20. Dyamenahalli K, Garg G, Shupp JW, Kuprys PV, Choudhry MA, Kovacs EJ. Inhalation injury: unmet clinical needs and future research. J Burn Care Res. 2019;40(5):570–84.
21. Romanowski KS, Palmieri TL, Sen S, Greenhalgh DG. More than one third of intubations in patients transferred to burn centers are unnecessary: proposed guidelines for appropriate intubation of the burn patient. J Burn Care Res. 2016;37(5):e409–14.
22. Rida J, Bouchriti Y, Ait Haddou M, Achbani A, Sine H, Serhane H. Meteorological factors and climate change impact on asthma: a systematic review of epidemiological evidence. J Asthma. 2024;61(12):1601–10.
23. Tan YQ, Cao LF, Shen J, Yu Y. Climatic factors correlate with innate immune response in children with Dermatophagoides farinae-induced allergic asthma. J Int Med Res. 2012;40(2):740–7.
24. Tham KW, Zuraimi MS, Koh D, Chew FT, Ooi PL. Associations between home dampness and presence of molds with asthma and allergic symptoms among young children in the tropics. Pediatr Allergy Immunol. 2007;18(5):418–24.
25. Hayes D Jr, Jhaveri MA, Mannino DM, Strawbridge H, Temprano J. The effect of mold sensitization and humidity upon allergic asthma. Clin Respir J. 2013;7(2):135–44.
26. Kim JH, Hyong IH. Analysis of changes in pulmonary functions at rest following humidity changes. J Phys Ther Sci. 2015;27(4):1063–5.
27. Aitken ML, Marini JJ, Culver BH. Humid air increases airway resistance in asthmatic subjects. West J Med. 1988;149(3):289–93.
28. Zuo YY, Acosta E, Policova Z, Cox PN, Hair ML, Neumann AW. Effect of humidity on the stability of lung surfactant films adsorbed at air-water interfaces. Biochim Biophys Acta. 2006;1758(10):1609–20.
29. Wolkoff P, Azuma K, Carrer P. Health, work performance, and risk of infection in office-like environments: the role of indoor temperature, air humidity, and ventilation. Int J Hyg Environ Health. 2021;233:113709.
30. Anderson SD, Kippelen P. A proposal to account for the stimulus, the mechanism, and the mediators released in exercise-induced bronchoconstriction. Front Allergy. 2023;4:1004170.
31. Parsons JP, Hallstrand TS, Mastronarde JG, Kaminsky DA, Rundell KW, Hull JH, et al. An official American Thoracic Society clinical practice guideline: exercise-induced bronchoconstriction. Am J Respir Crit Care Med. 2013;187(9):1016–27.
32. McFadden ER Jr, Lenner KA, Strohl KP. Postexertional airway rewarming and thermally induced asthma. New insights into pathophysiology and possible pathogenesis. J Clin Invest. 1986;78(1):18–25.
33. Deal EC Jr, McFadden ER Jr, Ingram RH Jr, Jaeger JJ. Hyperpnea and heat flux: initial reaction sequence in exercise-induced asthma. J Appl Physiol Respir Environ Exerc Physiol. 1979;46(3):476–83.
34. Gilbert IA, McFadden ER Jr. Airway cooling and rewarming. The second reaction sequence in exercise-induced asthma. J Clin Invest. 1992;90(3):699–704.
35. Smith CM, Anderson SD. Hyperosmolarity as the stimulus to asthma induced by hyperventilation? J Allergy Clin Immunol. 1986;77(5):729–36.
36. Aitken ML, Marini JJ. Effect of heat delivery and extraction on airway conductance in normal and in asthmatic subjects. Am Rev Respir Dis. 1985;131(3):357–61.
37. Argyros GJ, Phillips YY, Rayburn DB, Rosenthal RR, Jaeger JJ. Water loss without heat flux in exercise-induced bronchospasm. Am Rev Respir Dis. 1993;147(6 Pt 1):1419–24.
38. Ingenito E, Solway J, Lafleur J, Lombardo A, Drazen JM, Pichurko B. Dissociation of temperature-gradient and evaporative heat loss during cold gas hyperventilation in cold-induced asthma. Am Rev Respir Dis. 1988;138(3):540–6.
39. Hallstrand TS, Moody MW, Aitken ML, Henderson WR Jr. Airway immunopathology of asthma with exercise-induced bronchoconstriction. J Allergy Clin Immunol. 2005;116(3):586–93.

40. Murphy RC, Lai Y, Nolin JD, Aguillon Prada RA, Chakrabarti A, Novotny MV, et al. Exercise-induced alterations in phospholipid hydrolysis, airway surfactant, and eicosanoids and their role in airway hyperresponsiveness in asthma. Am J Physiol Lung Cell Mol Physiol. 2021;320(5):L705–l14.
41. D'Amato M, Molino A, Calabrese G, Cecchi L, Annesi-Maesano I, D'Amato G. The impact of cold on the respiratory tract and its consequences to respiratory health. Clin Transl Allergy. 2018;8:20.
42. Andersen ZJ, Vicedo-Cabrera AM, Hoffmann B, Melén E. Climate change and respiratory disease: clinical guidance for healthcare professionals. Breathe (Sheff). 2023;19(2):220222.
43. Chen X, Zhu T, Wang Q, Wang T, Chen W, Yao Y, et al. Higher temperature and humidity exacerbate pollutant-associated lung dysfunction in the elderly. Environ Res. 2024;245:118039.
44. Lepeule J, Litonjua AA, Gasparrini A, Koutrakis P, Sparrow D, Vokonas PS, et al. Lung function association with outdoor temperature and relative humidity and its interaction with air pollution in the elderly. Environ Res. 2018;165:110–7.
45. Areal AT, Singh N, Zhao Q, Berdel D, Koletzko S, von Berg A, et al. The influence of short-term weather parameters and air pollution on adolescent airway inflammation. Int J Environ Res Public Health. 2023;20(19)
46. Rice MB, Li W, Wilker EH, Gold DR, Schwartz J, Zanobetti A, et al. Association of outdoor temperature with lung function in a temperate climate. Eur Respir J. 2019;53(1):1800612.
47. Mekhuri S, Quach S, Barakat C, Sun W, Nonoyama ML. A cross-sectional survey on the effects of ambient temperature and humidity on health outcomes in individuals with chronic respiratory disease. Can J Respir Ther. 2023;59:256–69.
48. Han A, Deng S, Yu J, Zhang Y, Jalaludin B, Huang C. Asthma triggered by extreme temperatures: from epidemiological evidence to biological plausibility. Environ Res. 2023;216(Pt 2):114489.
49. Liao W, Zhou L, Zhao X, Song L, Lu Y, Zhong N, et al. Thermoneutral housing temperature regulates T-regulatory cell function and inhibits ovalbumin-induced asthma development in mice. Sci Rep. 2017;7(1):7123.
50. Jaakkola K, Saukkoriipi A, Jokelainen J, Juvonen R, Kauppila J, Vainio O, et al. Decline in temperature and humidity increases the occurrence of influenza in cold climate. Environ Health. 2014;13(1):22.
51. Vignola AM, Chanez P, Polla BS, Vic P, Godard P, Bousquet J. Increased expression of heat shock protein 70 on airway cells in asthma and chronic bronchitis. Am J Respir Cell Mol Biol. 1995;13(6):683–91.
52. Hayes D Jr, Collins PB, Khosravi M, Lin RL, Lee LY. Bronchoconstriction triggered by breathing hot humid air in patients with asthma: role of cholinergic reflex. Am J Respir Crit Care Med. 2012;185(11):1190–6.
53. Mirsaeidi M, Motahari H, Taghizadeh Khamesi M, Sharifi A, Campos M, Schraufnagel DE. Climate change and respiratory infections. Ann Am Thorac Soc. 2016;13(8):1223–30.
54. Lin S, Luo M, Walker RJ, Liu X, Hwang SA, Chinery R. Extreme high temperatures and hospital admissions for respiratory and cardiovascular diseases. Epidemiology. 2009;20(5):738–46.
55. O'Lenick CR, Cleland SE, Neas LM, Turner MW, McInroe EM, Hill KL, et al. Impact of heat on respiratory hospitalizations among older adults in 120 large US urban areas. Ann Am Thorac Soc. 2024.
56. Zwicker D, Ostilla-Mónico R, Lieberman DE, Brenner MP. Physical and geometric constraints shape the labyrinth-like nasal cavity. Proc Natl Acad Sci U S A. 2018;115(12):2936–41.

Chapter 2
Breathing While at Depth

Kay Tetzlaff

Introduction

Exposure to the underwater environment requires humans to either dive while holding their breath or dive with breathing support. Breathing at depth can be technically enabled by use of a self-contained underwater breathing apparatus (SCUBA) or surface- or underwater habitat-based supply systems that deliver the breathing gas through pressure hoses to the diver's helmet or mask. Of these alternatives, SCUBA diving is, by far, the most common underwater diving activity with an estimated 2.5 million participants in the USA in 2024 [1]. Breath-hold diving, although restricted by individual breath-hold endurance, has gained traction more recently as a competitive sports activity, with athletes competing in several underwater disciplines.

The underwater environment poses unique challenges to the respiratory system, due to the effects of immersion in water and the physical effects elicited on gases by increased pressure. Both hypoxia and hyperoxia may stress the respiratory system when freediving or breathing gas at depth, respectively. Exposure to elevated nitrogen pressure may cause narcosis and increase the risk of unconsciousness and drowning, while decompression stress arising from tissue saturation at depth may result in decompression sickness (DCS). Rapid changes in ambient pressure may cause barotrauma of gas-filled cavities such as the lungs, and increased work of breathing combined with augmented cardiac filling may precipitate immersion pulmonary edema and cardiac failure.

This chapter aims to provide an overview of the physiologic challenges to the respiratory system when diving with an underwater breathing apparatus or diving

---

K. Tetzlaff (✉)
Department of Sports Medicine, University Hospital Tübingen, Tübingen, Germany
e-mail: Kay.tetzlaff@klinikum.uni-tuebingen.de

E. R. Swenson, A. M. Luks (eds.), *The Lungs at the Extremes of Environment and Age*, Respiratory Medicine, https://doi.org/10.1007/978-3-031-98371-9_2

on a single breath-hold. The underlying pathologic mechanisms of these unique diving-related hazards will be reviewed, with an emphasis on pulmonary physiology and pathophysiology at depth.

The Underwater Environment

Basic SCUBA equipment consists of a cylinder containing compressed breathing gas at high pressure, a demand-valve regulator, and a buoyancy control device holding the equipment on the diver's back. The regulator reduces the high-pressure breathing gas in the cylinder to ambient pressure and supplies gas on demand at depth. Most commonly, atmospheric air is utilized as breathing gas. However, other gas mixtures with varying nitrogen concentrations such as "Enriched Air Nitrox," in which the fractional concentration of oxygen exceeds 21%, or pure oxygen may be utilized for special diving purposes. For deep sea diving, gas mixtures different than air may be used with distinct inert gases such as helium replacing nitrogen, to alleviate the work of breathing and risk of narcosis at high pressures.

Pressure

Diving is associated with exposure to higher-than-normal atmospheric pressure, since ambient pressure at depth is a function of the water column acting on the body and the atmospheric sea level pressure. Sea level pressure or one atmosphere absolute (ata) is equivalent to the pressure of a column of 760 mm of mercury or 759.75 mmHg. When diving, pressure increases with depth; for every 10 m, pressure increases by approximately 1 ata (Table 2.1).

According to *Pascal's law*, pressure exerted at any point on a confined liquid is transmitted uniformly in all directions, so that body tissue volume will not change. Although pressure per se does not affect liquidous body tissues, effects on the

Table 2.1 Pressure-depth equivalents and gas density while breathing air at depth

	Depth		Ambient pressure		O_2 partial pressure	N_2 partial pressure	Gas density
	m	feet	ata	mmHg	mmHg	mmHg	
Sea level	0	0	1	757.5	1.575	5.925	1×
	10	33	2	1,515	3.15	11.85	2×
	20	66	3	2,272.5	4.725	17.775	3×
	30	98	4	3,030	6.3	23.7	4×
	40	123	5	3,787.5	7.875	29.625	5×

O_2 oxygen, *N_2* nitrogen, *ata* atmospheres absolute

neurological system have been reported at depths beyond 100–150 m, a situation referred to as *high pressure nervous syndrome*.

Since pressure and volume are inversely proportional at constant temperature according to *Boyle's law*, a given gas volume will shrink with increasing water depth. Conversely, gas will expand with decreasing pressure upon ascent from depth. For a gas mixture such as atmospheric air, according to *Dalton's law*, the fractional concentrations of each gas in that mixture remain the same, independent of pressure. The partial pressure of each component gas is dependent on its fractional concentration and total pressure. The fractional concentration of oxygen in air is 0.21, and at normal atmospheric pressure, the partial pressure of oxygen (pO_2) is 157.5 mmHg. At a depth of 30 m with an ambient pressure of 4 ata, the fractional concentration of oxygen is still 0.21; however, the partial pressure of oxygen (pO_2) is 630 mmHg.

Temperature changes are proportional to gas volume according to *Charles' law*. Thus, gas volume inside the cylinder as well as inside the buoyancy device may expand with increasing temperature. Exposing diving gear to the sun and heat should therefore be avoided after filling with gas at the surface.

Submersion

Beyond the increase in ambient pressure, water submersion has other important effects on human performance. Water is about 800 times denser than air at sea level, which increases the energy cost of locomotion and reduces exercise efficiency in the underwater environment. The density of water also affects a diver's buoyancy. According to *Archimedes' principle*, an object partially or wholly immersed in a fluid is buoyed up by a force equal to the weight of the fluid displaced by the object. The diver's total density depends upon incompressible tissues and the volume and density of highly compressible gas stores carried within the body (e.g., the lungs). Inflating or deflating the buoyancy device helps the diver maintain neutral buoyancy to avoid sinking or floating; inspired and expired lung volume while breathing also affects buoyancy at depth. As buoyancy is dependent on the density of the liquid, divers in fresh water need less weight to sink from the surface as the upward buoyant force is lower than salty sea water.

The higher density of water results in approximately 15 times higher thermal conductivity compared to atmospheric air. Heat loss in ambient atmospheric air is mainly governed by radiation and convection. When submersed in water, thermoneutrality—the temperature at which there is no heat transfer between the water and the body—ranges from 30 to 36 °C. Since the temperature of seawater is usually well below the thermoneutral temperature for humans, divers are at risk of hypothermia and, thus, suitable protection is needed to reduce heat loss through convection, evaporation, and respiration. As water temperature decreases and time passes, metabolism increases in proportion to the drop in skin and core temperatures.

Conversely, in water that is above the thermoneutral temperature, there is a significant risk of hyperthermia. Given these circumstances, hypothermia, hyperthermia, and heat stroke are serious hazards that can result from prolonged submersion and physical exercise in the underwater environment.

Immersion of the face causes a measurable decrease in heart rate and cardiac output, a phenomenon referred to as the *diving response*. This response is initiated by peripheral vasoconstriction via cutaneous receptors of the trigeminal nerve around the nose and mouth through a cutaneous-visceral parasympathetically mediated reflex. In addition to immersion, apnea, hypoxia, and other factors alone or in combination can trigger the diving response.

Immersion in water neutralizes the pressure gradient between the lower and upper half of the body, resulting in the redistribution of about 700–1000 mL of blood from extremities into the thorax [2]. The resulting increase in cardiac output enhances pulmonary blood flow, thereby increasing pulmonary vascular blood volume and pressure. Engorgement of the pulmonary capillaries reduces the compliance of the lung. Vital capacity is reduced by approximately 10–15% while residual volume (RV) is increased by 7% [3]. Cardiac output increases according to the water level of immersion in the erect posture; the reported 32–62% increase in cardiac output is due to increased stroke volume, which counteracts the decrease in heart rate [4]; mean arterial pressure is unchanged. Increased right heart end-diastolic volume increases myocardial wall tension and atrial stretching, which augments release of the diuretically-acting atrial natriuretic peptide, resulting in the so-called *divers' diuresis*.

Respiratory Mechanics at Depth

The density of a given gas is directly proportional to the pressure the gas is under at a specific temperature and volume; as volume changes with ambient pressure, density changes accordingly. The density of atmospheric air doubles at a depth of 10 m, and triples at 20 m, etc. Since air supplied by the SCUBA regulator at depth is subject to ambient pressure, ventilated air is denser compared to sea level pressure. For example, when breathing air at 30 m, where total ambient pressure is 4 ata, the gas density is four times higher compared to sea level. Higher gas density causes more turbulent airflow throughout conducting airways, increasing airway resistance and, as a result, the work of breathing. Accordingly, maximal expiratory flow is inversely proportional to the square root of gas density, which has been shown experimentally for maximal voluntary ventilation (MVV) and forced expiratory volume in one second (FEV_1) [5]. At 30 m, MVV and FEV_1 are reduced by 50% of the respective measured values at sea level. To reduce the respiratory resistance of breathing gas mixtures at greater depths, helium–oxygen is usually used instead of nitrogen–air when diving deeper than 50–60 m.

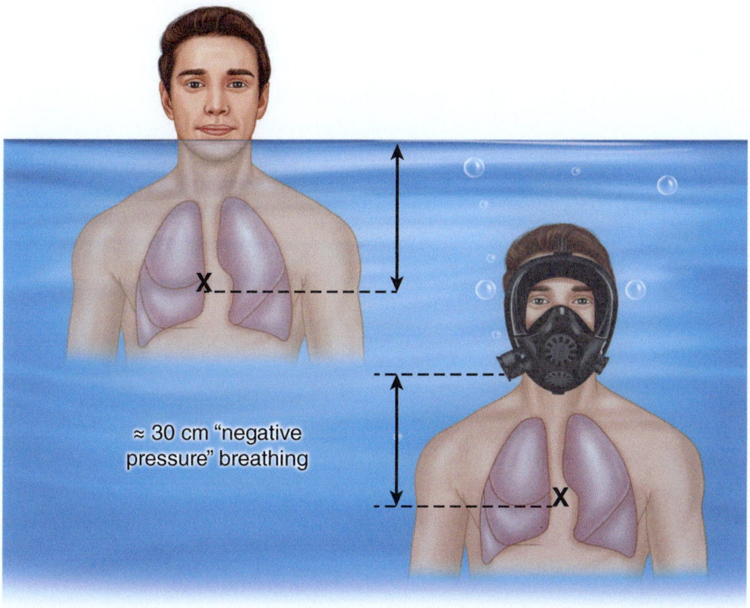

Fig. 2.1 Illustration of negative pressure breathing when immersed up to the neck in water (left side) or fully submersed in water and breathing from SCUBA in an upright position (right side)

Breathing at depth is further impeded by elastic load and dead space of the SCUBA equipment, adding to the increased work of breathing at depth. Diving gear, such as wetsuits and weight belts, may aggravate the restrictive force on the chest wall and abdomen, particularly if the equipment is excessively tight. Further, the effects of negative pressure breathing caused by compression of the chest increase the effort of breathing because of the external hydrostatic pressure, creating a greater transpulmonary pressure difference. During diving, when the open diving regulator is held at the mouth, negative-pressure breathing occurs with static lung loading when the breathing regulator is at a different hydrostatic pressure than the lung centroid, impacting the force required by the inspiratory muscles (Fig. 2.1). Elevated static lung loading may adversely impact breathing efficiency, causing respiratory muscle fatigue and dyspnea at depth [6].

In summary, a combination of resistive and elastic loading is largely responsible for the reduction in exercise ventilation at depth; the airways resistance component of this increase in work of breathing depends upon depth (Table 2.2). Increased respiratory load and work of breathing are associated with the risk of reduced alveolar ventilation and hypercarbia, which can lead to life-threatening physical and mental status changes for divers, including, in the worst case, unconsciousness [7].

Table 2.2 Factors challenging the airways while breathing at depth

Gas density ↑[a]
Resistance of the breathing regulator ↑
SCUBA dead space ↑
Static lung loading
Tightly fitting neoprene suit
Exercise (e.g., swimming against an underwater current)
Breathing cold and dry gas while mouth breathing

[a] Density increases proportional to depth, i.e., breathing becomes more difficult the deeper the dive

Blood Gases at Depth

Breathing air at increased ambient pressure increases the arterial partial pressure of oxygen (PaO_2) according to ambient pressure and the inspired fraction of oxygen (F_IO_2). Measurements of arterial blood gases at distinct depths during simulated dives have confirmed that the true increases in PaO_2 correspond to those predicted from the respective ambient pressure [8].

While oxygen is vital to sustain life, cellular and biochemical effects induced by breathing molecular oxygen at elevated partial pressures are potentially harmful. Pulmonary oxygen toxicity has long been known to occur at longer-duration exposure to pO_2 greater than 375 mmHg, e.g., breathing air with an F_IO_2 greater than 0.50 at atmospheric pressure. However, oxygen may exert toxic effects on other systems of the body including the eyes, red blood cells, liver, heart, kidneys, and endocrine system. Acute toxicity to the central nervous system, as indicated by immediate onset of nausea, numbness, dizziness, twitching, hearing and visual disturbances, unconsciousness, and convulsions, has been reported to occur with pO_2 greater than 1,050 mmHg [9]. This partial pressure would be reached at a depth of 4 m when diving with a closed-circuit underwater rebreathing apparatus using 100% oxygen as breathing gas. When SCUBA diving and breathing air at depth, the critical pO_2 of 1,050 mmHg is reached at approximately 57 m. Thus, divers using oxygen rebreathers or enriched air nitrox breathing gas mixtures need to carefully plan their dive to avoid exceeding a certain maximum diving depth. Of note, susceptibility to oxygen toxicity has a high interpersonal and intra-individual variability, necessitating even more conservative dive planning.

The arterial partial pressure of carbon dioxide ($PaCO_2$) is more variable, with some studies reporting mild hypocapnia at depth and others demonstrating no changes or mild hypercapnia. Unlike oxygen, which is supplied at increasing partial pressures at depth, alveolar ventilation is typically tightly regulated to maintain $PaCO_2$ of approximately 40 mmHg and remains constant for a given workload, irrespective of depth. However, increased work of breathing at depth may cause spontaneous or voluntary hypoventilation (routinely practiced by some divers to save breathing gas), resulting in CO_2 retention. The extent of workload, water temperature, and body position at depth may account for variations in $PaCO_2$ measured during simulated dives. Of note, hyperoxia attenuates the ventilatory response to hypercapnia and has been shown to decrease ventilation during exercise [10].

Since atmospheric air contains approximately 78% nitrogen, 21% oxygen, and small amounts of other gases, the partial pressure of nitrogen (PN_2) increases with ambient pressure at depth. In contrast to oxygen, nitrogen is inert and not metabolized by the tissues. Since it is relatively insoluble in blood, the arterial PN_2 rapidly equilibrates with the alveolar PN_2. However, nitrogen molecules dissolve in body tissues until equilibration between the tissue and ambient PN_2, according to *Henry's law*, which states that the solubility of a gas in a liquid is directly proportional to the partial pressure of the gas above that liquid.

Elevated tissue PN_2 exerts direct effects on the central nervous system that have been described as inert gas narcosis [11]. Breathing compressed air at 30 m with an equivalent PN_2 of 2,625 mmHg invariably results in signs of nitrogen narcosis such as minor cognitive impairment. At depths greater than 30–50 m, more apparent symptoms resembling those of alcohol or marijuana intoxication occur, with the severity of these symptoms increasing with depth. As with alcohol, there is some interindividual and intraindividual variability of onset and severity of inert gas narcosis. Risk factors that can affect an individual's susceptibility to narcosis include fatigue, exercise, water temperature, anxiety, and hypercapnia. Different inert gases show distinct narcotic potency, which is related to the lipophilic properties of the respective gas. As the brain and nervous system have an especially high lipid content, uptake of excess nitrogen by lipids in these tissues causes swelling in cell membranes, leading to dysregulation of cell surface proteins. Disruption of gamma-aminobutyric acid neurotransmission has also been considered a possible mechanism. Inert gas narcosis is an acute response to high partial pressure and, as a result, the effects are rapidly alleviated by reduction of the partial pressure of the inert gas, i.e., ascending in case of breathing air at depth. However, there is evidence that indicates some of the symptoms persist until the end or after the dive [12]. Since the narcotic potency of helium or hydrogen is much lower than that of nitrogen, replacing nitrogen with less narcotic inert gases is preferred for deep dives.

Decompression Stress and Venous Gas Embolism

When breathing air at depth, nitrogen dissolves in body tissues in proportion to the PN_2 of the air inspired at the respective ambient pressure. The volume of dissolved nitrogen in blood and tissues increases until equilibrium with the gas phase is achieved, at which point the tissue is saturated with nitrogen. Saturation follows a pressure gradient that is determined by the difference between the ambient PN_2 and a tissue's PN_2. Saturation kinetics can be described by a first-order exponential function where nitrogen uptake in the blood and other tissues is mainly dependent on the pressure gradient, temperature, and inherent tissue characteristics such as tissue perfusion (Fig. 2.2). Thus, the rate of nitrogen uptake varies across distinct

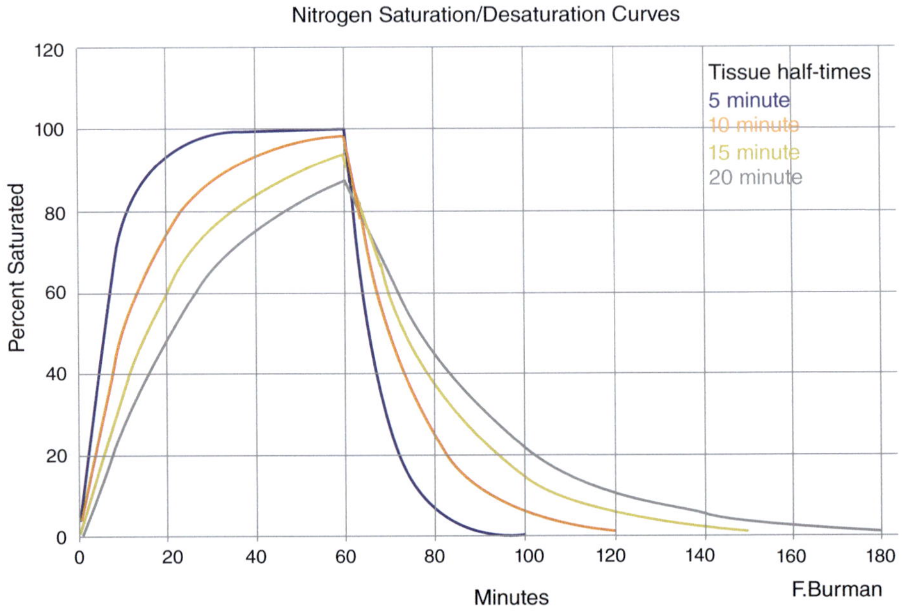

Fig. 2.2 Illustration of nitrogen saturation and washout curves for body tissues with distinct (slower and faster) saturation kinetics

body tissues with so-called "fast" and "slow" tissues such as the blood and adipose tissue, respectively, showing distinct saturation kinetics [13].

During the decompression phase of a dive, ambient pressure falls when ascending from depth. This decompression eventually creates a pressure gradient between tissue PN_2 and alveolar PN_2 such that nitrogen molecules leave solution and form free gas, depending on the pressure gradient, temperature, and tissue characteristics. Gas phase formation may be de novo or through growth from preexisting gas-filled voids in liquids called gas micronuclei. Critical tissue supersaturation may arise when tissue PN_2 sufficiently exceeds ambient PN_2. Nitrogen microbubbles form within supersaturated tissue and then continue to grow if the surrounding tissue is sufficiently supersaturated. This high gas supersaturation is required to overcome the *Laplace* pressure at the point of transition from dissolved gas to a nitrogen bubble. Generation of a PN_2 gradient sufficient to cause supersaturation depends on decompression time (i.e., the ascent rate from depth) [14, 15]. Early observations on experimental decompressions of goats saturated to depths of 50 m showed that limiting decompression time to half the ambient pressure reduced decompression sickness, leading to *Haldane's* concept of tissues' halftimes. This became the basis for modern decompression algorithms, limiting critical tissue supersaturation during ascent from depth. Decreasing ambient pressure during ascent will rapidly equilibrate arterial and alveolar $PN_{2,}$ and arterial tissue perfusion will establish a gradient for outward diffusion of nitrogen, enabling washout and elimination through venous return. While fast tissues may equilibrate with inspired PN_2 almost immediately, slow tissues continue to eliminate nitrogen throughout the ascent from depth and even after surfacing and reaching atmospheric ambient pressure.

Most dives result in the formation of gas microbubbles that predominantly originate in systemic veins and are carried away by the bloodstream to the pulmonary circulation, where they are eliminated. Venous nitrogen emboli are easily detected by Doppler ultrasound or echocardiography after SCUBA dives [16]. Using two-dimensional ultrasound, the size of emboli was estimated to range between 20 and 40 μm on average, although larger emboli up to 700 μm have been detected in a canine model of decompression sickness [17]. In humans, venous gas emboli typically appear within 15 min of surfacing from depth and may continue to appear for several hours post-dive. Venous gas emboli have frequently been detected after SCUBA dives and are commonly observed in the absence of any clinical signs or symptoms [18–20]. Usually, these venous gas emboli are trapped in the pulmonary capillary bed and eventually eliminated by diffusion into the alveolar space. Accordingly, venous gas emboli may elicit acute respiratory responses such as a decrease in diffusion capacity for carbon monoxide (DL_{CO}) [21], which correlates with the burden of venous gas emboli [22].

The capacity of the lung to filter gas emboli depends on the size and rate of bubbles trapped in the pulmonary circulation. The overload threshold of the pulmonary vasculature in a canine model was identified at an infusion rate of 0.3 mL kg^{-1} min^{-1} [23, 24]. Rates higher than 0.35 mL kg^{-1} min^{-1} increased pulmonary artery pressure, and arterial gas emboli could be detected by Doppler ultrasound in >50% of animals. Further studies confirmed these findings, showing that significant decompression stress resulted in an increased risk of a spillover of venous gas emboli to the arterial circulation, and the occurrence of gas bubbles in the left atrium followed the time-course and amount of venous gas emboli [25, 26]. However, arterial gas emboli have been detected in asymptomatic humans after otherwise uneventful and conservative SCUBA dives, suggesting passage of venous gas emboli through right-to-left shunts [20, 27]. A patent foramen ovale has experimentally been shown to allow gas passage during decompression [28], but extracardiac shunts such as intrapulmonary arterio-venous anastomoses may also account for gas passage in divers without a foramen ovale [29]. However, the occurrence of venous gas emboli after SCUBA dives is highly variable even during comparable dive profiles (e.g., depth, ascent rate, etc.), which has been attributed to high within-subject variability in gas embolism grades [30].

Diving-Related Injury

The unique environmental challenges when breathing at depth put the diver at risk for unique injury (Table 2.3). Lung injury may be caused by rapid pressure changes during decompression from depth, resulting in pulmonary barotrauma or

Table 2.3 Physiological challenges and associated health risks/hazards during a SCUBA dive

SCUBA Dive	Physiological challenge	Health risk/hazard
Descent from surface	Diving response	Bradycardia
	Central blood pooling Work of breathing ↑	Pulmonary edema
	Nitrogen uptake	Narcosis
Bottom phase	Hyperoxia	O_2 Toxicity
	Alveolar Hypoventilation and CO_2 Retention	Unconsciousness
Ascent from depth	Nitrogen washout	Decompression sickness Arterial gas embolism (via right-to-left shunt)
	Intrapulmonary gas expansion	Pulmonary barotrauma Arterial gas embolism Pneumothorax Interstitial emphysema

decompression illness (DCI). Also, individual susceptibility to the effects of exercise while below the surface of the water may result in diving-related pulmonary edema. Although serious injury is uncommon, elucidating the pathophysiological mechanisms of diving-related acute lung injury is important to better understand associated risk factors and how injury can be prevented.

Decompression Illness

Injury caused by the pathological effects of excess gas in blood or tissue during or after reduction in ambient pressure falls under the heading of decompression illness [31, 32], which encompasses two pathophysiologically distinct medical conditions, decompression sickness and arterial gas embolism.

Decompression sickness (DCS) refers to symptoms and signs caused by decompression stress or, in other words, the generation of intracorporeal inert gas bubbles. While the presence of venous gas emboli poorly predicts DCS, inert gas emboli may exert pathological effects when distorting surrounding tissue and damaging cells. Intravascular air emboli have been shown to cause hypoxemia and hemodynamic changes, including increased pulmonary artery pressure and pulmonary vascular resistance [33–35]. Humoral and cellular changes include activation of the complement system and leukocytes [36, 37], inducing proinflammatory cascades that result in hemoconcentration and leakage through the vascular endothelium [38, 39]. The magnitude of these changes correlates with the rate and volume of venous gas emboli, with lower bubble numbers less likely to produce hypoxemia or gross hemodynamic and/or fluid abnormalities. Clinical manifestations of DCS depend on the mechanical and biochemical effects of gas bubbles in situ and range from musculoskeletal pain to severe neurological injury with paralysis of limbs. Mild DCS can be due to mechanical irritation of tendon sheaths or joint capsules when inert gas bubbles form within these inhomogeneously perfused tissue compartments. Gas bubbles may be transferred to or grow within the bone marrow, causing a rise in intermedullary pressure, which is supported by the observation that DCS limb/joint or muscle pain, historically called *the bends*, is immediately responsive to recompression in most cases. DCS can also present as pruritus and rash, which is thought to be due to endothelial damage to the skin with blood extravasation from cutaneous vessels. While the presence of *livedo racemosa* due to thrombo-embolic obstruction of skin arterioles and capillaries strongly supports the diagnosis of DCS, skin manifestations are not required to diagnose DCS. Severe DCS is characterized by neurological signs and symptoms and is due to particular nitrogen saturation and elimination kinetics of the nervous tissues and its short ischemia tolerance. Neurological injury is presumed to be due to the thrombogenic effect of venous gas bubbles in the epidural venous plexus surrounding the spinal cord, causing venous stasis and spinal cord ischemia. Common neurological symptoms include numbness, tingling, paresthesia, and abnormal sensation and typically progress from mild paresthesia to regional numbness and weakness, and later paresis of the affected limbs. Symptoms usually occur within hours after decompression, but in severe cases, they may present shortly after the dive. A rare but severe manifestation of DCS is *respiratory decompression sickness*, which is caused by a heavy burden of nitrogen gas emboli in the pulmonary circulation. Typical symptoms of what is often referred to as the chokes include tachypnea, cough, cyanosis, and thoracic discomfort or pain. In a canine model of DCS pulmonary hypertension, systemic hypotension, hemoconcentration, and hypoxia occurred [40]. Pathological findings include pulmonary edema in the setting of normal left ventricular end-diastolic pressure. The authors postulated that microvascular permeability was altered by venous bubble emboli formed during decompression. In sheep, it could be shown that the amount of lung microvascular injury could be controlled by the rate of venous gas embolism and was reversible within 1–2 days [39]. When decompression from depth was followed by simulated exposure to high altitiude, an increased mean pulmonary artery pressure following the detection of high precordial bubble grades corresponded with the onset of restlessness and respiratory difficulty [41]. These studies showed that massive embolization of the pulmonary capillary bed precipitates respiratory decompression sickness. While common SCUBA dive profiles usually prevent massive nitrogen gas embolization, the incidence of respiratory decompression sickness in aviators has been reported as high as 6% [42].

Exposure to high altitude will elevate the risk of DCS after diving, due to lower barometric pressure compared to sea level. When SCUBA diving in a lake at high altitude, decompression times and stops must be adjusted for altitude, since N_2 saturation in water will be comparable to a dive in sea water. However, when surfacing from a freshwater dive at high altitude, ambient pressure will be lower than sea level pressure and, thus, require more decompression time to eliminate N_2 from body tissues. Common dive algorithms used for sea diving need to be adapted when diving at high altitude, and diving should be delayed after arriving at a dive site at a higher altitude. This will allow the nitrogen absorbed in the body to equilibrate to the lower ambient pressure. Another altitude-related mechanism of DCS risk increase is exposure to high altitude after SCUBA diving at sea level. A reduction in cabin pressure during commercial air travel to an equivalent altitude of approximately 2400 m will increase N_2 supersaturation in body tissues that have not completed N_2 washout when flying after diving, which may worsen existing DCS symptoms or precipitate DCS in a previously asymptomatic diver [43]. Therefore, in most recreational diving scenarios, a 24-h preflight surface interval is recommended to allow for complete N_2 elimination from body tissues after diving.

Arterial gas embolism (AGE) is caused by the entry of gas into the pulmonary veins or directly into the arteries of the systemic circulation. When breathing air at depth, gas may enter the arteries because of pulmonary barotrauma due to overexpansion of the lung during ascent from depth, or as a result of paradoxical embolism of venous nitrogen bubbles. Paradoxical embolism occurs when the gas bubbles traverse a right-to-left shunt, such as a pulmonary arteriovenous malformation, or because the venous bubble burden is so high that the pulmonary capillary beds cannot clear the gas into the alveoli fast enough. When free air enters the pulmonary vasculature and is carried to the heart and arterial circulation, serious injury may result. Air bubbles can reach the brain, occlude blood vessels, and cause stroke-like events within minutes of surfacing from a SCUBA dive. The most common signs and symptoms of arterial gas embolism are neurologic. A stroke-like syndrome with unilateral neurological symptoms has been considered typical for diving-related AGE. However, a more atypical presentation with bilateral symptoms may also be seen and therefore does not exclude AGE. The symptoms of *cerebral arterial gas embolism* develop suddenly. The clinical presentation, however, is determined by the absolute quantity of gas and the affected areas of the brain, and may range from minor motor weakness and headache to hemiparesis, convulsions, and loss of consciousness. Time to onset of symptoms may be delayed, and initial improvement may occur even without therapy, secondary to partial clearance of air emboli. Magnetic resonance imaging (MRI) may demonstrate focal lesions in the brain after arterial gas embolism [44]. AGE can mimic decompression sickness, and the presentation of the two syndromes of decompression illness may be clinically indistinguishable due to overlap in neurological signs in symptoms. Also, both may develop simultaneously in some patients. Treatment of AGE consists of basic or advanced cardiac life support, administration of 100% oxygen, rehydration, and transport to a recompression facility where oxygen will then be administered at increased ambient pressure.

A *patent foramen ovale (PFO),* the most common right-to-left shunt, has been demonstrated to be another risk factor for decompression illness in divers [45–47]. The prevalence of a patent foramen ovale among the diving population equals that of the total population [19, 45]. Meta-analysis of three studies that investigated incidence for decompression illness and echocardiographic presence of a PFO in different diving populations revealed a 2.6-fold increase in the risk for DCS/DCI [48]. The incidence of DCS in that population averaged 0.02%. More recent data from a large perspective study in 148 divers and 66,859 collected dives reported 8.3% of divers without and 28.6% of divers with a right-to-left shunt experiencing DCS/DCI during the study period [49], indicating incidences per 10,000 dives of 1.95 and 5.16, respectively with an overall relative risk of 2.65 (CI 1.05–6.72). The size of PFO has been shown to be related to the risk of DCI, with a 4.4-fold risk increase in divers with grade 2 PFO and a 6.6-fold increase in divers with grade 3 PFO [50]. PFO closure may successfully prevent future DCS/DCI in scuba divers with a high-grade PFO [51], but the risk of DCI may remain even after PFO closure [52]. A risk stratification strategy may be as effective as PFO closure in reducing DCI incidence for divers with low-grade PFO but not high-grade PFO [53].

Pulmonary Barotrauma

Breathing gas may enter the pulmonary veins through rupture of alveolar or bronchiolar structures when transpulmonary pressure increases during ascent from depth. According to *Boyle's law*, intrapulmonary gas will expand when ambient pressure decreases and may lead to overdistension of airway or alveolar structures if the decrease in pressure (i.e., the ascent rate) exceeds the rate at which the expanding gas can escape through the airways. Closure of the upper airways by, for example, breath-holding or airflow limitation due to pulmonary pathology may precipitate this pathophysiology.

Unprotected dogs with trachea closed that were rapidly decompressed from ambient pressures of 2,297.25 or 4,594.5 mmHg, equivalent to depths of about 31 and 62 m, developed pulmonary barotrauma when the intratracheal pressure reached a critical level of approximately 80.25 mmHg [54]. This could be prevented by the application of thoraco-abdominal binders, despite a rise in intratracheal pressure to levels of 180 mmHg. Accordingly, experiments with fresh unchilled human cadavers showed that lung barotrauma occurred at intrapulmonary pressures of about 72.75–80.25 mmHg [55]. Binding of both the chest and abdomen required much higher pressures of 132.75–189.75 mmHg. It was further observed that rupture of the visceral pleura occurred where basal pleural adhesions were present.

Pulmonary barotrauma may cause breathing gas to track along the perivascular sheaths of the pulmonary arteries and erupt into such an artery or move toward the hilum on expiration and dissect into the thin-walled pulmonary veins. Gas can also dissect toward the lung periphery, rupturing into the pleural space, causing *pneumothorax*, or escaping gas may track into the peribronchial space or mediastinum, causing interstitial or mediastinal emphysema [54]. Furthermore, extra-alveolar gas can also pass through the esophageal hiatus and enter the peritoneum and cause *pneumoperitoneum* [56, 57]. When air is entering the left atrium, upright position during ascent, buoyancy, and blood flow dynamics may favor the distribution of gas bubbles to the brain, causing *cerebral arterial gas embolism*. Accordingly, serious injury often presents as a stroke-like syndrome with unilateral neurological symptoms [13, 58]. However, a more atypical presentation with bilateral neurologic symptoms has been reported [59]. Cognitive symptoms and unconsciousness are most frequently present, while seizures, focal motor deficits, visual disturbances, vertigo, and sensory changes can also be seen [60, 61]. Symptoms will generally present immediately after surfacing or even during ascent.

Lung parenchymal abnormalities and airflow limitation due to obstructive airway diseases increase the risk of pulmonary barotrauma. Poorly ventilated structures such as blebs, bullae, or cysts can cause air trapping [62–64] (Fig. 2.3), and valve mechanisms of emphysematous changes have been described, explaining obstruction of the outflow of gas from the alveolar spaces during exhalation [65]. In a few cases, proof could be presented that small peripheral bullae noted on chest computed tomography (CT) during diagnostic evaluation had been present before the injury [66, 67]. Because of the common misconception that serious decompression illness does not occur at shallow depth, it is worth emphasizing that, in fact, the

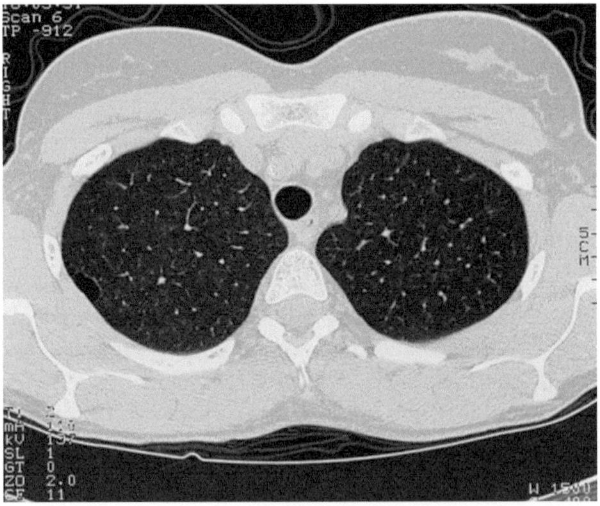

Fig. 2.3 Chest CT of a 35-year-old female dive master who performed two open sea SCUBA dives to 35 m (115 ft) and 37 m (121 ft), respectively, with a short surface interval of only 90 min. After surfacing from the second dive, she was unable to get onto the dive boat and complained about chest pain and a cough. She had right-sided hemiparesis and became temporarily unconscious. A livedo racemosa could be observed on her trunk and thighs. She was administered 100% oxygen via face mask and transferred to a hyperbaric treatment facility; symptoms had improved already when arriving at the facility. Her history was remarkable for a spontaneous pneumothorax 7 years before the diving accident. A right-to-left shunt was found by contrast echocardiography. CT of the chest revealed subpleural bullae in the right lung—apical and lateral in the middle lobe. A diagnosis of decompression illness was made, with clinical signs of decompression sickness and probable arterial gas embolism through a patent foramen ovale. It remained unclear whether the lung bullae were incidental or had caused arterial gas embolism following lung barotrauma. The patient fully recovered following hyperbaric oxygen therapy

risk for pulmonary barotrauma is greatest just below the surface, since the ambient pressure doubles between the water surface and 10 m, with the relative change in volume being greatest at that depth range. Accordingly, cases of arterial gas embolism have been reported during shallow water SCUBA dives in a swimming pool [68–70].

Diving-Related Pulmonary Edema

Diving-related pulmonary edema, often referred to as immersion pulmonary edema, has been more widely recognized over the past two decades. Initially observed in SCUBA divers [47], it can also be seen in swimmers, snorkelers, triathletes, freedivers, and during aqua jogging [71–74]. The clinical presentation includes shortness of breath, cough, hemoptysis, with chest tightness or pain reported less frequently [75]. Clinical investigation reveals hypoxemia, tachypnea, and crackles on lung exam [76, 77]. Radiographs and computerized tomography scans of the lungs demonstrate infiltrates and patchy acinar and lobular ground-glass and consolidative opacities. These findings are typically bilateral, but unilateral edema has been reported [76] such as in military trainees swimming in a lateral decubitus position, with radiographic findings in the dependent, submersed lung [78]. Clinical symptoms usually resolve within 24–48 h with removal from water, supportive treatment, and oxygen administration [79]. However, dyspnea and cough can persist for several days after the incident [80]. The incidence of immersion pulmonary edema is lower in males (0.09%) compared to females (0.75%) and increase with age [79]; however, incidences of up to 5% were reported among members of the military special forces, a group that tends to be relatively young relative to the general population [73, 81].

The pathophysiology of immersion pulmonary edema is multifactorial, with immersion in water and individual susceptibility playing a pivotal role in its development. Immersion redirects blood into the thorax, thereby raising central blood volume and hence cardiac filling pressures. Exercise in water further increases thoracic blood volume and left atrial, pulmonary artery, and capillary pressures [82]. However, mean pulmonary artery pressure during immersion varies widely between individuals, indicating the possibility of interindividual differences in susceptibility. It could be shown that mean pulmonary artery pressure in single individuals rose above the threshold for pathological values during submaximal exercise but not during dry exercise [83]. While there was an ameliorative effect of oxygen during immersed exercise in thermoneutral water [84], hyperoxia did not protect against increased pulmonary artery pressures associated with immersed exercise in cold [85]. Subjects with a history of immersion pulmonary edema developed higher mean pulmonary artery pressure and pulmonary artery wedge pressure during exercise in cold water in comparison with the general population [86], and these pressures could be reduced with a single 50-mg oral dose of sildenafil, a phosphodiesterase type 5 (PDE5) inhibitor.

In contrast to swimming-induced pulmonary edema, however, physical exercise was not a contributing factor in reported cases of SCUBA diving-related immersion pulmonary edema [87–90]. Increased accumulation of extravascular lung water without development of clinical signs of pulmonary edema could be detected in healthy individuals after repetitive deep SCUBA dives without physical exercise [89]. Accumulation of extravascular lung water was associated with significantly increased mean pulmonary artery pressure, decreased left ventricular contractility, and an augmented N-terminal pro-B-type natriuretic peptide (NT-proBNP) release, suggesting significant cardiopulmonary strain. Increased internal and external breathing resistances and static lung loading may facilitate the development of lung edema, and augment intrathoracic pressure swings between inspiration and expiration, and greater negative intrathoracic pressure during inspiration will increase right ventricular preload. It has been shown that negative pressure breathing combined with exercise resulted in much greater increases in right heart preload, pulmonary artery systolic pressure, and worsened interstitial edema formation as demonstrated by lung ultrasound [91]. Divers with a history of immersion pulmonary edema exhibit higher inspiratory workload, and it was speculated that this was due to more pronounced impairment of pulmonary compliance induced by immersion [92].

Breath-Hold Diving

Breath-hold or freediving shares the exposure to the underwater environment with SCUBA diving, i.e., the effects of water immersion and higher ambient pressure on human physiology. However, the individual's breath-hold endurance will usually determine the underwater exposure when freediving. Since breath-hold time in normal untrained subjects is around 1–2 min, freedives are usually of rather short duration and will not reach greater depths. Trained competitive freedivers, however, can hold their breath for on average 5 min [93] and reach depths exceeding 100 m on a single breath-hold.

Breath-hold endurance is affected by several factors such as starting lung volume, metabolic rate, and the decrease in blood oxygen levels as well as the buildup of carbon dioxide. The human *diving response* is an important physiologic mechanism to reduce oxygen consumption and is elicited by apnea and face immersion. It is characterized by a synergistic sympathetic and parasympathetic activation and catecholamine increase, redistribution of blood flow to maintain adequate oxygen supply to hypoxia-sensitive organs, and reduced heart rate. The diving response is highly variable and can be modified by physiological as well as emotional factors. Elite freedivers have developed certain adaptations to repeated apnea training, such as greater tolerance to hypoxia and hypercapnia, and a more pronounced diving response. The oxygen-sparing effect has been shown to be proportional to the degree of the bradycardia [94].

When freediving, the lungs are subject to gas compression according to Boyle's law. For example, at 10 m depth, the intrathoracic gas volume will have shrunk to half of its normal volume. Accordingly, the alveolar pO_2 and PCO_2 will increase with increasing water depth. Since the mixed venous partial pressures do not change, both gases diffuse increasingly into the blood with a corresponding increase in arterial partial pressures. The arterial pO_2 is about 250 mmHg when reaching a depth of 20 m [95]. Paradoxically, the compression-related increased alveolar PCO_2 leads to a transfer of CO_2 from the alveolus into the blood during descent. Due to the high CO_2 solubility, however, the immersion-related increase in intrathoracic blood volume with consecutive increase in pulmonary blood flow leads to a redistribution of CO_2 into the well-perfused tissues of the organism. During ascent, the alveolar pO_2 also decreases again and can reach the mixed-venous value. This can lead to paradoxical diffusion of O_2 from the blood into the alveolar space, which further intensifies the body's reduced supply of oxygen and can lead to dangerous hypoxia during ascent from greater depths.

Compression of the lungs stresses pulmonary physiology when the total intrathoracic gas volume reaches the residual volume (RV) during descent. Below this volume, the negative airway pressure may lead to an influx of blood and fluid into the alveolar space. According to a classical physiological concept, the ratio of total lung capacity (TLC) to RV was considered the limiting factor for deep diving in apnea. Accordingly, a diver with a given TLC of 6 L and an RV of 1.5 L (TLC/RV ratio of 4:1) would reach the RV at a depth of 30 m. However, immersion-related redistribution of blood into the thoracic cavity will mitigate the risk of *negative pressure barotrauma* (lung squeeze) and allow trained breath-hold divers to safely reach greater depths [2].

Competitive elite freedivers use a breathing technique called *glossopharyngeal insufflation*, also known as "lung-packing," to further increase their available lung volume. This will reduce the risk of negative pressure pulmonary barotrauma by increasing the TLC/RV ratio and enlarging available oxygen stores. The breathing technique consists of maximum inhalation up to the TLC and, after closing the larynx, pressing air into the trachea by opening the larynx. This swallowing maneuver is repeated several times, and measured increases in TLC between 22% and 50% have been reported, accompanied by intra- and transpulmonary pressures that can reach values of 80 and 109 cmH_2O, respectively [96, 97]. Glossopharyngeal insufflation must overcome lung recoil pressure to increase lung volume above TLC, and a transient decline of lung elastic recoil could be confirmed by a gradual decline of static compliance over 5 min even when subjects had exhaled and returned to tidal breathing [98]. Glossopharyngeal insufflation is mainly used only in extreme freediving to achieve longer breath-hold endurance or reach greater depths. Complications inherent to this technique include loss of consciousness due to the massive acute reduction in cardiac output and venous return, as well as pulmonary overdistension and barotrauma. In a series of computed tomography examinations after subjects performing these maneuvers, asymptomatic air pockets in the mediastinum were detected in several cases [99].

Hypoxic disorders of the central nervous system (blackouts) as well as hypoxia of the muscles (loss of motor control) are among the most common clinical complications of extreme competitive freediving [100, 101]. Blackout and loss of consciousness are serious complications as they will lead to drowning underwater if the freediver is unattended. Development of critical hypoxia during freediving is usually prevented by an urgency to breathe, the breath-hold breaking point, where arterial PCO_2 exceeds approximately 45–55 mmHg and involuntary inspiratory efforts such as contractions of the thorax and the diaphragm occur [102, 103]. However, several mechanisms may manipulate the timely occurrence of the breathing stimulus and, thus, increase the risk of shallow water blackout. Hyperventilation before diving will lower carbon dioxide in blood, hence extend the time until reaching the threshold value to trigger breathing. Extreme hyperventilation may decrease arterial PCO_2 to a critically low level at the beginning of the breath-hold dive. With prolonged breath-hold duration, pO_2, however, continues to decrease and may cause cerebral hypoxia towards the end of a breath-hold dive, when the rising PCO_2 as the main respiratory drive has not yet reached the hypercarbia level needed to trigger breathing.

Another mechanism increasing the risk of blackout when freediving is an accelerated fall in pO_2 during ascent from greater depth. At depth, hyperoxia prevails due to thoracic gas compression, so that the increasing arterial PCO_2 remains as the sole respiratory stimulus. During ascent from a deep breath-hold dive, arterial pO_2 falls more steeply due to declining ambient pressure and continued oxygen consumption, which may even be worsened by paradoxical diffusion of oxygen from tissues and blood into the alveolar space. Unconsciousness will occur when the rising PCO_2 has not yet reached the breath-stimulating threshold.

Although it has been considered unlikely that freedivers would accumulate enough nitrogen to provoke *decompression sickness*, there have been early reports from commercial sea harvesting freedivers of a neurological syndrome (*Taravana*) with rapid onset of partial paralysis, visual problems, difficulties with hearing or speech, and even cases of loss of consciousness. The main clinical manifestations are cerebral, including stroke and cognitive impairment. Japanese Ama breath-hold divers perform repeated dives up to 30 m depth for 1–2 min duration with surface rests of about 1 min before the next dive, in working shifts of 2–4 h. According to Haldane's decompression theory, N_2 release is slower than uptake, so that repeated breath-hold dives with short surface intervals can lead to the accumulation of N_2 in the tissue. Indeed, the repetitive dive pattern of the Korean Ama breath-hold divers has been found to generate hypernitrogenemia [104]. Corresponding clinical symptoms and neuroimaging findings have been reported from early experimental studies [105] and neuroimaging studies in commercial Japanese breath-hold divers [106]. Apart from clinical pathology findings, proof of intravascular gas bubbles by Doppler measurements in professional Japanese breath-hold divers after a series of repetitive dives to depths of 20 m were reported [107], and tear film bubble formation was demonstrated in submarine escape tank divers after repeated breath-hold dives to 30 m [108]. There have been reports of neurological symptoms after only few repeated breath-hold dives to 45 m depth presenting with paralysis of the limbs, and a case of speech disturbance and amnesia after a final single free dive to 90 m

[109], and a stroke-like syndrome in a young and healthy freediver after four dives to about 100 m depth [110]. At greater depths, very high diffusion gradients between the alveolar PN_2 and tissue PN_2 nitrogen will diffuse forcefully from the alveolar space. It has also been calculated that human lungs are highly efficient at gas exchange just prior to total collapse [111], and N_2 uptake will increase linearly during descent up to that point. The ascent from great depth does not allow for longer decompression stops, which may enable N_2 microgas bubbles to form in body tissues. It remains unclear, however, whether N_2 gas bubbles may form directly in the cerebral arteries or if venous bubbles may shunt through a foramen ovale or intrapulmonary arteriovenous anastomosis [106]. Hypoxia could promote the recruitment of an intrapulmonary arteriovenous anastomosis, allowing venous N_2 bubbles to pass into the arterial circulation [112]. However, neuroradiological imaging is supporting an alternative hypothesis of in situ formation of autochthonous bubbles in the cerebral capillaries, with reversible involvement of blood-brain barrier/endothelial dysfunction in DCS according to posterior reversible encephalopathy syndrome [113, 114].

Conclusion

Diving poses unique and significant challenges to human physiology. Underwater performance and safety are influenced by several factors, including immersion, exposure to water, the limitations of breath-hold endurance, variations in ambient pressure, the effects of breathing gases at elevated ambient pressure, the use of breathing apparatus, and sensory impairment. Injury can occur due to unsafe diving practices or preexisting medical risks. Although rare, serious injury is often related to respiratory conditions and includes pulmonary barotrauma, noncardiogenic pulmonary edema, or hemoptysis. Breathing air under increased ambient pressure may cause narcosis and decompression illness due to inadequate elimination of dissolved nitrogen when pressure decreases. A comprehensive understanding of the pathophysiology, injury patterns, and treatment protocols for both common and life-threatening diving injuries is essential for advising, diagnosing, and treating recreational divers. Many physicians lack adequate training to identify or manage dive-related injuries. Understanding diving risks is vital for preventing these injuries when assessing medical fitness.

References

1. DEMA Diving Equipment and Marketing Association. 2024 Diving Fast Facts. 2024. https://www.dema.org/store/download.aspx?id=7811b097-8882-4707-a160-f999b49614b6. Accessed 30 Jan 2025.
2. Schaefer KE, Allison RD, Dougherty JH, Carey CR, Walker R, Yost F, Parker D. Pulmonary and circulatory adjustments determining the limits of depth in breathhold diving. Science. 1968;162:1020–3.

3. Girandola RN, Wiswell RA, Mohler JG, Romero GT, Barnes WS. Effects of water immersion on lung volumes: implications for body composition analysis. J Appl Physiol. 1977;43(2):276–9. https://doi.org/10.1152/jappl.1977.43.2.276. PMID: 893282.
4. Pendergast DR, Lundgren CE. The underwater environment: cardiopulmonary, thermal, and energetic demands. J Appl Physiol. 2009;106(1):276–83. https://doi.org/10.1152/japplphysiol.90984.2008.
5. Maio DA, Farhi LE. Effect of gas density on mechanics of breathing. J Appl Physiol. 1967;23:687–93.
6. Thalmann ED, Sponholtz DK, Lundgren CE. Effects of immersion and static lung loading on submerged exercise at depth. Undersea Biomed Res. 1979;6(3):259–90.
7. Dunworth SA, Natoli MJ, Cooter M, Cherry AD, Peacher DF, Potter JF, Wester TE, Freiberger JJ, Moon RE. Hypercapnia in diving: a review of CO_2 retention in submersed exercise at depth. Undersea Hyperb Med. 2017;44(3):191–209. https://doi.org/10.22462/5.6.2017.1.
8. Paganini M, Moon RE, Boccalon N, Melloni GEM, Giacon TA, Camporesi EM, Bosco G. Blood gas analyses in hyperbaric and underwater environments: a systematic review. J Appl Physiol. 2022;132(2):283–93. https://doi.org/10.1152/japplphysiol.00569.2021.
9. Harabin AL, Survanshi SS, Homer LD. A model for predicting central nervous system oxygen toxicity from hyperbaric oxygen exposures in humans. Toxicol Appl Pharmacol. 1995;132:19–26. https://doi.org/10.1006/taap.1995.1082.
10. Pirnay F, Marechal R, Dujardin R, Lamy M, Deroanne R, Petit JM. Exercise during hyperoxia and hyperbaric oxygenation. Int Z Angew Physiol. 1973;31(4):259–68. https://doi.org/10.1007/BF00693711.
11. Bennett PB, Dossett AN. Mechanism and prevention of inert gas narcosis and anaesthesia. Nature. 1970;228(5278):1317–8. https://doi.org/10.1038/2281317a0.
12. Balestra C, Lafere P, Germonpre P. Persistence of critical flicker fusion frequency impairment after a 33 mfw SCUBA dive: evidence of prolonged nitrogen narcosis? Eur J Appl Physiol. 2012;112:4063–8.
13. Bove AA. Diving medicine. Am J Respir Crit Care Med. 2014;189(12):1479–86. https://doi.org/10.1164/rccm.201309-1662CI.
14. Carturan D, Boussuges A, Vanuxem P, Bar-Hen A, Burnet H, Gardette B. Ascent rate, age, maximal oxygen uptake, adiposity, and circulating venous bubbles after diving. J Appl Physiol. 2002;93:1349–56.
15. Eckenhoff RG, Olstad CS, Carrod G. Human dose-response relationsship for decompression and endogenous bubble formation. J Appl Physiol. 1990;69:914–8.
16. Blogg SL, Gennser M, Møllerløkken A, Brubakk AO. Ultrasound detection of vascular decompression bubbles: the influence of new technology and considerations on bubble load. Diving Hyperb Med. 2014;44(1):35–44.
17. Hills BA, Butler BD. Size distribution of intravascular air emboli produced by decompression. Undersea Biomed Res. 1981;8:163–70.
18. Dunford RG, Vann RD, Gerth WA, Pieper CF, Huggins K, Wacholtz C, et al. The incidence of venous gas emboli in recreational diving. Undersea Hyperb Med. 2002;29:247–59.
19. Glen SK, Georgiadis D, Grosset DG, Douglas JDM, Lees KR. Transcranial Doppler ultrasound in commercial air divers: a field study including cases with right-to-left shunting. Undersea Hyperb Med. 1995;22:129–35.
20. Ljubkovic M, Dujic Z, Møllerløkken A, Bakovic D, Obad A, Breskovic T, Brubakk AO. Venous and arterial bubbles at rest after no-decompression air dives. Med Sci Sports Exerc. 2011;43(6):990–5. https://doi.org/10.1249/MSS.0b013e31820618d3.
21. Dujic Z, Eterovic D, Denoble A, Krstacic G, Tocilj J, Gosovic S. Effect of a single air dive on pulmonary diffusing capacity in professional divers. J Appl Physiol. 1993;74:55–61.
22. Thorsen E, Risberg J, Segadal K, Hope A. Effects of venous gas microemboli on pulmonary gas transfer function. Undersea Hyperb Med. 1995;22:347–53.
23. Butler BD, Hills BA. The lung as a filter for microbubbles. J Appl Physiol. 1979;47:537–43.

24. Butler BD, Hills BA. Transpulmonary passage of venous air emboli. J Appl Physiol. 1985;59:543–7.
25. Reuter M, Tetzlaff K, Brasch F, Gerriets T, Weiher M, Struck N, et al. Computed chest tomography in an animal model for decompression sickness: radiologic, physiologic, and pathologic findings. Eur Radiol. 2000;10:534–41.
26. Vik A, Brubakk AO, Hennessy TR, Jessen BM, Ekker M, Slørdahl SA. Venous air embolism in swine: transport of gas bubbles through the pulmonary circulation. J Appl Physiol. 1990;69:237–44.
27. Gerriets T, Tetzlaff K, Liceni T, Schafer C, Rosengarten B, Kopiske G, et al. Arteriovenous bubbles following cold water sport dives: relation to right-to-left shunting. Neurology. 2000;55:1741–3.
28. Ries S, Knauth M, Kern R, Klingmann C, Daffertshofer M, Sartor K, et al. Arterial gas embolism after decompression: correlation with right-to-left shunting. Neurology. 1999;52:401–4.
29. Ljubkovic M, Zanchi J, Breskovic T, Marinovic J, Lojpur M, Dujic Z. Determinants of arterial gas embolism after scuba diving. J Appl Physiol. 2012;112:91–5.
30. Doolette DJ, Murphy FG. Within-diver variability in venous gas emboli (VGE) following repeated dives. Diving Hyperb Med. 2023;53(4):333–9. https://doi.org/10.28920/dhm53.4.333-339.
31. Mitchell SJ, Bennett MH, Moon RE. Decompression sickness and arterial gas embolism. N Engl J Med. 2022;386(13):1254–64. https://doi.org/10.1056/NEJMra2116554.
32. Vann RD, Butler FK, Mitchell SJ, Moon RE. Decompression illness. Lancet. 2011;377(9760):153–64. https://doi.org/10.1016/S0140-6736(10)61085-9.
33. Bove AA, Hallenbeck JM, Elliott DH. Circulatory responses to venous air embolism and decompression sickness in dogs. Undersea Biomed Res. 1974;1:207–20.
34. Neuman TS, Spragg RG, Wagner PD, Moser KM. Cardiopulmonary consequences of decompression stress. Respir Physiol. 1980;41:143–53.
35. Peterson BT, Grauer SE, Hyde RW, Ortiz C, Moosavi H, Utell MJ. Response of pulmonary veins to increased intracranial pressure and pulmonary air embolization. J Appl Physiol. 1980;48:957–64.
36. Levin LL, Stewart GJ, Lynch PR, Bove AA. Blood and blood vessel wall changes induced by decompression sickness in dogs. J Appl Physiol. 1981;50:944–9.
37. Ward CA, McCullough D, Fraser WD. Relation between complement activation and susceptibility to decompression sickness. J Appl Physiol. 1987;62:1160–6.
38. Albertine JJ, Wiener-Kronish JP, Koike K, Staub NC. Quantification of damage by air emboli to lung microvessels in anesthetized sheep. J Appl Physiol. 1984;57:1360–8.
39. Ohkuda K, Nakahara K, Binder A, Staub NC. Venous air emboli in sheep: reversible increase in lung microvascular permeability. J Appl Physiol. 1981;51:887–94.
40. Catron PW, Flynn ET, Yaffe Y, Bradley ME, Thomas LB, Hinman D, et al. Morphological and physiological responses of the lungs of dogs to acute decompression. J Appl Physiol. 1984;57:467–74.
41. Atkins CE, Lehner CE, Beck KA, Dubielzig RR, Nordheim EV, Lanphier EH. Experimental respiratory decompression sickness in sheep. J Appl Physiol. 1988;65:1163–71.
42. Wirjosemito SA, Touhey JE, Worman WT. Type II altitude decompression sickness (DCS): U. S. Air Force experience with 133 cases. Aviat Space Environ Med. 1989;60:256–62.
43. Freiberger JJ, Denoble PJ, Pieper CF, Uguccioni DM, Pollock NW, Vann RD. The relative risk of decompression sickness during and after air travel following diving. Aviat Space Environ Med. 2002;73(10):980–4.
44. Reuter M, Tetzlaff K, Hutzelmann A, Fritsch G, Steffens JC, Bettinghausen E, Heller M. MR imaging of the central nervous system in diving-related decompression illness. Acta Radiol. 1997;38(6):940–4. https://doi.org/10.1080/02841859709172107.
45. Germonpré P, Dendale P, Unger P, Balestra C. Patent foramen ovale and decompression sickness in sports divers. J Appl Physiol. 1998;84:1622–6.

46. Moon RE, Camporesi EM, Kisslo JA. Patent foramen ovale and decompression sickness in divers. Lancet. 1989;1:513–4.
47. Wilmshurst PT, Nuri M, Crother A, Webb-Peploe NM. Cold-induced pulmonary oedema in scuba-divers and swimmers and subsequent development of hypertension. Lancet. 1989;1:62–5.
48. Bove AA. Risk of decompression sickness with patent foramen ovale. Undersea Hyperb Med. 1998;25:175–8.
49. Germonpré P, Lafère P, Portier W, Germonpré F-L, Marroni A, Balestra C. Increased risk of decompression sickness when diving with a right-to-left shunt: results of a prospective single-blinded observational study (The "Carotid Doppler" Study). Front Physiol. 2021;12:763408.
50. Torti SR, Billinger M, Schwerzmann M, Vogel R, Zbinden R, Windecker S, Seiler C. Risk of decompression illness among 230 divers in relation to the presence and size of patent foramen ovale. Eur Heart J. 2004;25(12):1014–20.
51. Honěk J, Šrámek M, Honěk T, Tomek A, Šefc L, Januška J, Fiedler J, Horváth M, Novotný Š, Veselka J. Patent foramen ovale closure is effective in divers: long-term results from the DIVE-PFO registry. J Am Coll Cardiol. 2020;76(9):1149–50.
52. Lee HJ, Lim DS, Kang YC. Recurrent decompression illness even after the closure of patent foramen ovale in a diver. JACC Case Rep. 2022;5:101687. https://doi.org/10.1016/j.jaccas.2022.101687. eCollection 2023 Jan 4.
53. Honěk J, Šrámek M, Honěk T, Tomek A, Šefc L, Januška J, Fiedler J, Horváth M, Novotný Š, Brabec M, Veselka J. Screening and risk stratification strategy reduced decompression sickness occurrence in divers with patent foramen ovale. JACC Cardiovasc Imaging. 2022;15(2):181–9. https://doi.org/10.1016/j.jcmg.2021.06.019.
54. Schaefer KE, McNulty WP, Carey C, Liebow AA. Mechanisms in development of interstitial emphysema and air embolism on decompression from depth. J Appl Physiol. 1958;13:15–29.
55. Malhotra MS, Wright HC. The effects of a raised intrapulmonary pressure on the lungs of fresh unchilled cadavers. J Pathol Bacteriol. 1961;82:198–202.
56. Oh ST, Kim W, Jeon HM, Kim JS, Kim KW, Yoo SJ, Kim EK. Massive pneumoperitoneum after scuba diving. J Korean Med Sci. 2003;18:281–3.
57. Schriger DL, Rosenberg G, Wilder RJ. Shoulder pain and pneumoperitoneum following a diving accident. Ann Emerg Med. 1987;16:1281–4.
58. Melamed Y, Shupak A, Bitterman H. Medical problems associated with underwater diving. N Engl J Med. 1992;326:30–5.
59. Collins JJ. An unusual case of air embolism precipitated by decompression. N Engl J Med. 1962;266:595–8.
60. Kizer KW. Dysbaric cerebral air embolism in Hawaii. Ann Emerg Med. 1987;16:535–41.
61. Leitch DR, Green RD. Pulmonary barotrauma in divers and the treatment of cerebral arterial gas embolism. Aviat Space Environ Med. 1986;57:931–8.
62. Mellem H, Emhjellen S, Horgen O. Pulmonary barotrauma and arterial gas embolism caused by an emphysematous bulla in a scuba diver. Aviat Space Environ Med. 1990;61:559–62.
63. Reuter M, Tetzlaff K, Warninghoff V, Steffens JC, Bettinghausen E, Heller M. Computed tomography of the chest in diving-related pulmonary barotrauma. Br J Radiol. 1997;70:440–5.
64. Toklu AS, Kiyan E, Aktas S, Cimsit M. Should computed chest tomography be recommended in the medical certification of professional divers? A report of three cases with pulmonary air casts. Occup Environ Med. 2003;60:606–8.
65. Zaugg M, Kaplan V, Widmer U, Bauman PC, Russi EW. Fatal air embolism in an airplane passenger with a giant intrapulmonary bronchogenic cyst. Am J Respir Crit Care Med. 1998;157:1686–9.
66. Germonpré P, Balestra C, Pieters T. Influence of scuba diving on asymptomatic isolated pulmonary bullae. Diving Hyperb Med. 2008;38(4):206–11.
67. Tetzlaff K, Reuter M, Leplow B, Heller M, Bettinghausen E. Risk factors for pulmonary barotrauma in divers. Chest. 1997;112:654–9.

68. Banham N, da Silva E, Lippmann J. Cerebral arterial gas embolism (CAGE) during open water scuba certification training whilst practising a controlled emergency swimming ascent. Diving Hyperb Med. 2023;53(4):345–50. https://doi.org/10.28920/dhm53.4.345-350. PMID: 38091595.
69. Friehs I, Friehs M, Friehs GB. Air embolism with bilateral pneumothorax after a five-meter dive. Undersea Hyperb Med. 1993;20:155–7.
70. Weiss LD, Van Meter KM. Cerebral air embolism in asthmatic scuba divers in a swimming pool. Chest. 1995;107:1653–4.
71. Miller CC, Calder-Becker K, Modave F. Swimming-induced pulmonary edema in triathletes. Am J Emerg Med. 2010;28:941–6.
72. Pons M, Blickenstorfer D, Oechslin E, et al. Pulmonary oedema in healthy persons during scuba-diving and swimming. Eur Respir J. 1995;8:762–7.
73. Weiler-Ravell D, Shupak A, Goldenberg I, Halpern P, Shoshani O, Hirschhorn G, et al. Pulmonary oedema and haemoptysis induced by strenuous swimming. Br Med J. 1995;311:361–2.
74. Wenger M, Russi EW. Aqua jogging-induced pulmonary oedema. Eur Respir J. 2007;30:1231–2.
75. Grünig H, Nikolaidis PT, Moon RE, Knechtle B. Diagnosis of swimming induced pulmonary edema: a review. Front Physiol. 2017;31(8):652. https://doi.org/10.3389/fphys.2017.00652. eCollection 2017.
76. Hårdstedt M, Seiler C, Kristiansson I, et al. Swimming-induced pulmonary edema: diagnostic criteria validated by lung ultrasound. Chest. 2020;158(4):1586–95.
77. Lund KL, Mahon RT, Tanen DA, Bakhda S. Swimming-induced pulmonary edema. Ann Emerg Med. 2003;41:251–6.
78. Mahon RT, Kerr S, Amundson D, Parrish JS. Immersion pulmonary edema in special forces combat swimmers. Chest. 2002;122:383–4.
79. Hårdstedt M, Kristiansson L, Seiler C, Braman Eriksson A, Sundh J. Incidence of swimming-induced pulmonary edema: a cohort study based on 47,600 open-water swimming distances. Chest. 2021;160(5):1789–98. https://doi.org/10.1016/j.chest.2021.06.034.
80. Kristiansson L, Seiler C, Lundeqvist D, Braman Eriksson A, Sundh J, Hårdstedt M. Symptom duration, recurrence, and long-term effects of swimming-induced pulmonary edema: a 30-month follow-up study. Chest. 2023;164(5):1257–67. https://doi.org/10.1016/j.chest.2023.06.041.
81. Volk C, Spiro G, Boswell G, et al. Incidence and impact of swimming-induced pulmonary edema on navy seal candidates. Chest. 2021;159(5):1934–41.
82. Wester TE, Cherry AD, Pollock NW, et al. Effects of head and body cooling on hemodynamics during immersed prone exercise at 1 ata. J Appl Physiol. 2009;106:691–700.
83. Kovacs G, Berghold A, Scheidl S, Olschewski H. Pulmonary arterial pressure during rest and exercise in healthy subjects: a systematic review. Eur Respir J. 2009;34:888–94.
84. Peacher DF, Pecorella SR, Freiberger JJ, et al. Effects of hyperoxia on ventilation and pulmonary hemodynamics during immersed prone exercise at 4.7 ata: possible implications for immersion pulmonary edema. J Appl Physiol. 2010;109(1):68–78.
85. Fraser JA, Peacher DF, Freiberger JJ, Natoli MJ, Schinazi EA, Beck IV, Walker JR, Doar PO, Boso AE, Walker AJ, Kernagis DN, Moon RE. Risk factors for immersion pulmonary edema: hyperoxia does not attenuate pulmonary hypertension associated with cold water-immersed prone exercise at 4.7 ATA. J Appl Physiol. 2011;110(3):610–8. https://doi.org/10.1152/japplphysiol.01088.2010.
86. Moon RE, Martina SD, Peacher DF, Potter JF, Wester TE, Cherry AD, Natoli MJ, Otteni CE, Kernagis DN, White WD, Freiberger JJ. Swimming-induced pulmonary edema: pathophysiology and risk reduction with sildenafil. Circulation. 2016;133:988–96.
87. Castagna O, de Maistre S, Schmid B, Caudal D, Regnard J. Immersion pulmonary oedema in a healthy diver not exposed to cold or strenuous exercise. Diving Hyperb Med. 2018;48(1):40–4.

88. Hampson NB, Dunford RG. Pulmonary edema of scuba divers. Undersea Hyperb Med. 1997;24:29–33.
89. Marinovic J, Ljubkovic M, Obad A, Breskovic T, Salamunic I, Denoble PJ, Dujic Z. Assessment of extravascular lung water and cardiac function in trimix SCUBA diving. Med Sci Sports Exerc. 2010;42(6):1054–61.
90. Slade JB, Hattori T, Ray CS, Bove AA, Cianci P. Pulmonary edema associated with scuba diving. Chest. 2001;120:1686–94.
91. Castagna O, Regnard J, Gempp E, et al. The key roles of negative pressure breathing and exercise in the development of interstitial pulmonary edema in professional male SCUBA divers. Sports Med Open. 2018;4(1):1.
92. Druelle A, Mouhat B, Zbitou O, Castagna O. Static immersion and negative static lung load-induced right ventricle systolic function adaptation: a risk factor for immersion pulmonary edema. Chest. 2024;166(3):532–43. https://doi.org/10.1016/j.chest.2024.03.042.
93. Hansel J, Solleder I, Gfroerer W, Muth CM, Paulat K, Simon P, Heitkamp HC, Niess A, Tetzlaff K. Hypoxia and cardiac arrhythmias in breath-hold divers during voluntary immersed breath-holds. Eur J Appl Physiol. 2009;105:673–8.
94. Lindholm P, Lundgren CEG. The physiology and pathophysiology of human breath-hold diving. J Appl Physiol. 2009;106:284–92.
95. Muth CM, Radermacher P, Pittner A, Steinacker J, Schabana R, Hamich S, Paulat K, Calzia E. Arterial blood gases during diving in elite apnea divers. Int J Sports Med. 2003;24:104–7.
96. Lindholm P, Nyren S. Studies on inspiratory and expiratory glossopharyngeal breathing in breath-hold divers employing magnetic resonance imaging and spirometry. Eur J Appl Physiol. 2005;94:646–51.
97. Loring SH, O'Donnell CR, Butler JP, Lindholm P, Jacobson F, Ferrigno M. Transpulmonary pressures and lung mechanics with glossopharyngeal insufflation and exsufflation beyond normal lung volumes in competitive breath-hold divers. J Appl Physiol. 2007;102:841–6.
98. Tetzlaff K, Scholz T, Walterspacher S, Muth CM, Metzger J, Roecker K, Sorichter S. Characteristics of the respiratory mechanical and muscle function of competitive breath-hold divers. Eur J Appl Physiol. 2008;4:469–75.
99. Chung SC, Seccombe LM, Jenkins CR, Frater CJ, Ridley LJ, Peters MJ. Glossopharyngeal insufflation causes lung injury in trained breath-hold divers. Respirology. 2010;15:813–7.
100. Fitz-Clarke J. Adverse events in competitive breath-hold diving. Undersea Hyperb Med. 2006;33:55–62.
101. Lindholm P. Loss of motor control and/or loss of consciousness during breath-hold competitions. Int J Sports Med. 2007;28:295–9.
102. Schagatay E, Andersson J. Diving response and apneic time in humans. Undersea Hyperb Med J. 1998;25:13–9.
103. Schagatay E, van Kampen M, Emanuelsson S, Holm B. Effects of physical and apnea training on apneic time and the diving response in humans. Eur J Appl Physiol. 2000;82:161–9.
104. Radermacher P, Falke KJ, Park YS, Ahn DW, Hong SK, Qvist J, Zapol WM. Nitrogen tensions in brachial vein blood of Korean ama divers. J Appl Physiol. 1992;73:2592–5.
105. Paulev P. Decompression sickness following repeated breath-hold dives. J Appl Physiol. 1965;20:1028–103.
106. Kohshi K, Tamaki H, Lemaître F, Morimatsu Y, Denoble PJ, Ishitake T. Diving-related disorders in commercial breath-hold divers (Ama) of Japan. Diving Hyperb Med. 2021;51(2):199–206. https://doi.org/10.28920/dhm51.2.199-206.
107. Lemaitre F, Kohshi K, Tamaki H, Nakayasu K, Harada M, Okayama M, Satou Y, Hoshiko M, Ishitake T, Costalat G, Gardette B. Doppler detection in ama divers of Japan. Wilderness Environ Med. 2014;25:258–62.
108. Sheard PW. Ocular tear film bubble formation after breath-hold diving. Undersea Hyperb Med. 2008;35:79–82.
109. Schagatay E. Predicting performance in competitive apnea diving. Part III: deep diving. Diving Hyperb Med. 2011;41:216–28.

110. Tetzlaff K, Schoppenthau H, Schipke JD. Risk of neurological insult in competitive deep breath-hold diving. Int J Sports Physiol Perform. 2017;12:268–71.
111. Fitz-Clarke JR. Lung compression effects on gas exchange in human breath-hold diving. Respir Physiol Neurobiol. 2009;165:221–8.
112. Schipke JD, Tetzlaff K. Why predominantly neurological decompression sickness in breath-hold divers? J Appl Physiol. 2016;120:1474–7.
113. Druelle A, Castagna O, Roffi R, Louge P, Faivre A, Blatteau JE. Taravana syndrome and posterior reversible encephalopathy syndrome: a microbubble hypothesis for neurological accidents in breath-hold divers. Front Physiol. 2024;15:1478650. https://doi.org/10.3389/fphys.2024.1478650. eCollection 2024.
114. Sánchez-Villalobos JM, Fortuna-Alcaraz ML, Serrano-Velasco L, Pujante-Escudero Á, Garnés-Sánchez CM, Pérez-Garcilazo JE, Olea-González A, Pérez-Vicente JA. Breath-hold diving-related decompression sickness with brain involvement: from neuroimaging to pathophysiology. Tomography. 2022;8(3):1172–83. https://doi.org/10.3390/tomography8030096.

Chapter 3
Breathing and Pulmonary Circulation at High Altitudes

Marc Moritz Berger

This chapter describes the role of central and peripheral chemoreceptors in regulating the hypoxic and hypercapnic ventilatory response and highlights changes in pulmonary gas exchange, pulmonary mechanics, and dynamics at high altitudes. In addition, the current state of knowledge on how breathing is altered during sleep at high altitudes is briefly addressed with a special focus on periodic breathing. Finally, the mechanisms and consequences of hypoxic pulmonary vasoconstriction (HPV), including the pathogenesis of high-altitude pulmonary edema (HAPE), are discussed, along with a brief overview of its prevention and therapy.

An increase in ventilation is one of the earliest and most important processes of acclimatization to high altitude. Referred to as the hypoxic ventilatory response (HVR), this hypoxia-induced increase in ventilation counteracts the drop in alveolar and arterial partial pressure of oxygen (PO_2) that occurs due to the nonlinear decrease in barometric pressure with increasing altitude. HVR helps maintain arterial oxygen content, and thereby the convective oxygen delivery to tissues and cells, as high as possible in situations with reduced oxygen supply. While ventilatory acclimatization does not maintain the arterial PO_2 at sea level values, particularly at the extremes of elevation, acclimatization protects against acute altitude illnesses and improves cognitive and submaximal exercise performance [1].

M. M. Berger (✉)
Department of Anesthesiology, Intensive Care Medicine, Emergency Medicine and Pain Therapy, RKH Hospital Ludwigsburg, Ludwigsburg, Germany

E. R. Swenson, A. M. Luks (eds.), *The Lungs at the Extremes of Environment and Age*, Respiratory Medicine, https://doi.org/10.1007/978-3-031-98371-9_3

Control of Breathing

The physiologic, rhythmic breathing cycle is generated by four respiratory centers in the brain stem. It is modulated by a complex respiratory network, particularly by central and peripheral chemoreceptors which are located in the ventrolateral surface of the medulla and in the carotid and aortic bodies, respectively (Fig. 3.1). The chemoreceptors play a crucial role in the fine-tuning of ventilation by detecting changes in the partial pressure of carbon dioxide (PCO_2), pH, and PO_2 to adjust breathing accordingly.

In healthy humans, at sea level, the effect of the central chemoreceptors on ventilation dominates over the effect of the peripheral chemoreceptors. The central chemoreceptors react to changes in PCO_2 and hydrogen (H^+) ion concentration in the extracellular fluid of the brain. Because the blood–brain barrier is highly permeable to dissolved CO_2, an increase in arterial PCO_2 (P_aCO_2) increases the H^+ ion concentration in the cerebrospinal fluid, resulting in an increase in ventilation. The peripheral chemoreceptors are primarily sensitive to the arterial PO_2 (P_aO_2) but, to a lesser extent, are also sensitive to changes in P_aCO_2 and H^+ ion concentration. Under physiologic conditions at sea level, the influence of peripheral chemoreceptors on ventilation is assumed to be additive to the central chemoreflex drive [2, 3], with a relative contribution of about one-third when compared to the importance of the central chemoreceptors [4]. The response to hypoxic conditions is driven by the peripheral chemoreceptors alone [5], so with ascent to higher altitudes, the contribution of the peripheral chemoreceptors on ventilation increases. Among the peripheral chemoreceptors, the carotid bodies are more important for acute HVR in humans and most animals than the aortic bodies.

Of note, HVR is mediated by changes in P_aO_2 rather than by changes in arterial oxygen content. Thus, hypoxemia stimulates HVR, wherease reduced cerebral blood flow does not. This makes physiological sense because an increase in ventilation would not improve tissue oxygenation in case of low cardiac output but would improve the tissue's oxygen supply in hypoxic conditions.

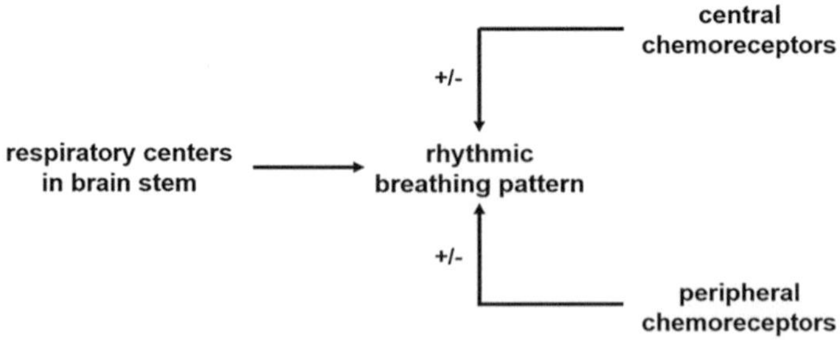

Fig. 3.1 Regulation of ventilation. The central and peripheral chemoreceptors are located in the ventrolateral surface of the medulla, and in the carotid and aortic bodies, respectively. At sea level, ventilation is modulated by about two-thirds by the central chemoreceptors and by about one-third by the peripheral chemoreceptors. For details, see text

Ventilation at High Altitudes

Upon ascent to high altitudes, ventilation increases, resulting in higher alveolar and arterial PO_2 and lower alveolar and arterial PCO_2 (Table 3.1). The fall in P_aCO_2 decreases central and peripheral chemoreceptor output, thereby acting as a negative feedback mechanism slowing the increase in ventilation.

The time course of HVR can best be characterized at rest with a given degree of hypoxia (Fig. 3.2). The HVR begins and stops immediately with the onset or removal of hypoxia [6], that is, it begins and ends within one breath of the detection of a change in P_aO_2 at the carotid body [5]. About 10 min later, a hypoxic ventilatory decline, the so-called "roll-off phenomenon" occurs [7]. Although the precise mechanism for the roll-off phenomenon is uncertain, it could result from the fall in P_aCO_2, decreased chemoreceptor sensitivity, increased cerebral blood flow, or other central nervous system inputs [8]. After about 30–60 min, ventilation increases again, eventually reaching a maximum after hours or even months, depending on the definite degree of hypoxia and the species [1, 6]. The physiological ventilatory responses that occur with acute exposure to hypoxia are generally referred to as ventilatory acclimatization to hypoxia (VAH) [9].

Significance of HVR at High Altitude

The hypoxia-induced increase in ventilation varies greatly in magnitude between healthy individuals by almost ten-fold. The increase in ventilation starts as the PO_2 falls and usually becomes more prominent once the inspired PO_2 is reduced to <100 mmHg [10], which corresponds to an altitude of about 3000 m or a $P_aO_2 < 60$ mmHg. At extremely high altitudes, where the ambient pressure—and thus the inspired PO_2—is significantly reduced, pronounced hyperventilation is a prerequisite to ensure a sufficiently high arterial PO_2. For example, in the absence

Table 3.1 Blood gases at low and high altitudes

	LA	HA day 1 evening	HA day 2 morning	HA day 2 Evening	HA day 3 morning	Altitude [m]
PO_2 [mmHg]	90 ± 11	54 ± 4	57 ± 4	57 ± 5	58 ± 4	3450
PCO_2 [mmHg]	35 ± 3	32 ± 3	31 ± 3	31 ± 2	30 ± 2	3450
PO_2 [mmHg]	84 ± 8	46 ± 5	48 ± 4	48 ± 5	49 ± 5	4559
PCO_2 [mmHg]	35 ± 3	28 ± 3	26 ± 2	26 ± 2	25 ± 2	4559

Data (mean ± SD) show the change in arterial or capillary PO_2 and PCO_2 at low altitudes and during the first 3 days at high altitudes. Values are combined from two studies at the Jungfraujoch (3450 m, upper lines, n = 78; [115, 116]) and two studies at the Capanna Regina Margherita (4559 m, lower lines, n = 56; [113, 117]). Of note, at altitudes equivalent to or close to the summit of Mount Everest (8848 m) the arterial PO_2 and PCO_2 have been reported to be about 25–30 mmHg and 8–13 mmHg, respectively [14–16]. *LA* low altitude (423 m), *HA* high altitude as indicated in the column on the far right

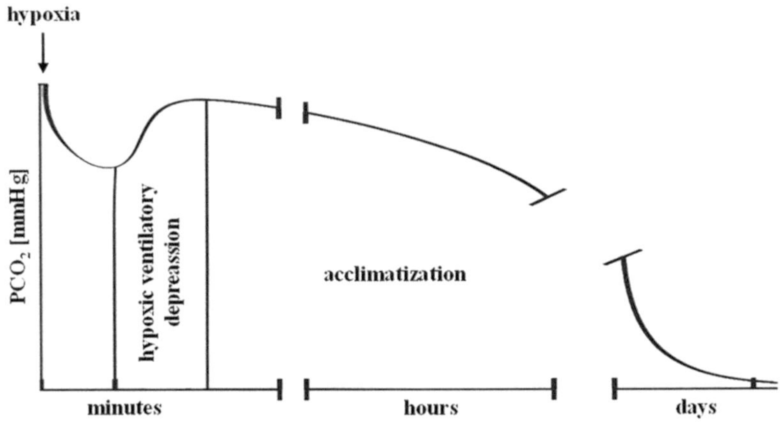

Fig. 3.2 Schematic illustration of the time course of the ventilatory response to a given degree of acute hypoxia. With the onset of hypoxia ventilation, i.e., breathing frequency and tidal volume, increase leading to a fall in alveolar and arterial PCO_2 [6]. After about 10 min a transient hypoxic ventilatory depression (roll-off phenomenon) occurs, before ventilation increases again. For details, see text. (Modified from [118])

of hyperventilation on the summit of Mount Everest, where the inspiratory PO_2 is only about 43 mmHg [11], the alveolar PO_2, as calculated by the alveolar gas equation with a respiratory exchange ratio of 0.8, would be −7 mmHg—a physiologically impossible value. It is only a strong ventilatory response that allows an individual to maintain an alveolar and arterial PO_2 sufficient to survive and perform physical work [12]. Under these conditions, extreme degrees of hyperventilation and respiratory alkalosis can be seen. During the 1981 American Medical Research Expedition to Everest, for example, the mean minute ventilation of a single mountaineer climbing for nearly 7 min at 8300 m was about 108 L/min with a respiratory rate of about 86 breaths/min [13]. Measurements taken during a simulated ascent of Mount Everest in a hypobaric chamber as well as measurements completed in mountaineers at or near the summit of Mount Everest have provided further evidence of the high degree of ventilation achieved at these altitudes with alveolar PCO_2 values ranging from 8 to 13 mmHg, which are sufficient to maintain a P_aO_2 of about 25–30 mmHg [14–16].

While it is generally assumed that a strong HVR is beneficial at extreme altitudes, excessive HVR may actually be a problem. Data collected during Mount Everest and K2 expeditions showed that climbers who reached these two summits without supplemental oxygen were characterized by a lower resting minute ventilation, breathing rate and ventilatory response to hypoxia, and a higher ventilatory reserve and ventilatory efficiency, compared to the climbers that were not successful or needed supplemental oxygen to reach the summit [17]. As an explanation, the authors suggested that individuals with a very strong, excessive HVR may reach their ventilatory limit already at lower altitudes, whereas those with a strong but not excessive HVR are able to sustain high levels of ventilation at extreme altitude while maintaining an adequate ventilatory reserve for the summit—particularly if relatively lower minute ventilation is compensated for by higher ventilatory efficiency [1, 17]. However, it is also possible that severe hypocapnia, resulting from extreme hyperventilation, led to cerebral vasoconstriction and reduced blood flow [18]. This may have decreased cerebral oxygen delivery with multifaceted potential consequences, including impaired cognitive [19] and psychomotor [20] performance.

HVR During Acclimatization

With arrival at high altitude, ventilatory acclimatization to hypoxia (VAH) starts as mirrored by an increase in minute ventilation. This increase is caused by an increased sensitivity of the peripheral chemoreceptors [21–23] that is reflected by a steepening of the HVR slope (i.e., the ventilation–SpO_2 response curve).

The majority of VAH takes place within the first 1–2 days at a given altitude [24], but depending on the absolute altitude attained and the ambient PO_2, it can take up to several weeks to complete [25]. For example, acclimatization may take about 4 days at 3000 m [10], 2–3 weeks at 4000 m [24], and around 4–6 weeks at 5050 m [26]. For altitudes over 8000 m, ventilatory acclimatization may take up to 11 weeks [25]. Following ventilatory acclimatization, ventilatory depression may occur in some long-term residents who have spent several years at altitude [27], but this response is likely influenced by age, altitude, and environmental and genetic factors [8], as well as by further adaptations at the microcirculatory and cellular/mitochondrial levels that improve O_2 delivery and the efficiency of O_2 utilization.

After returning to low altitude, the increased HVR persists for several days or weeks due to a sustained increased sensitivity of the peripheral chemoreceptors [21]. The exact duration depends on the duration and the height of the previous high-altitude exposure as well as on individual factors. Increased HVR aids acclimatization if the individual reascends soon again to high altitude [28].

Hypercapnic Ventilatory Response (HCVR)

As with HVR, the ventilatory response to CO_2 evolves over time and influences ventilatory acclimatization. In particular, the sensitivity of the central chemoreceptor response to CO_2 increases with prolonged stay at high altitudes [21, 22], such that the increase in ventilation for a given increase in P_aCO_2 is larger at high altitudes than would be the case at lower elevations [29]. This resetting of the hypercapnic ventilatory response (HCVR) is caused by a leftward shift and steepening of the ventilation–CO_2 response curve [30] that, in part, results from the reduction of bicarbonate ions (HCO_3^-) in the brain's extracellular fluid and the neuronal tissue as a result of renal compensation for the sustained respiratory alkalosis at high altitude

[31, 32]. The result is a reduced buffering capacity in the central compartment that increases the relative stimulation of central chemoreceptors by H^+ ions for a given PCO_2 [8].

Gas Exchange

The decrease in barometric pressure at high altitudes has significant effects on gas exchange. The reduction in alveolar PO_2 decreases the pressure gradient for the diffusion of oxygen across the alveolar–capillary membrane (i.e., the difference between alveolar and mixed venous PO_2). This slows the rate of diffusion and extends the time required for equilibration between the alveolar and capillary PO_2. Another factor delaying equilibration is the lower mixed venous PO_2 that increases blood O_2 solubility [33]. As long as an individual remains at rest, red blood cells remain in the pulmonary capillaries long enough to achieve full equilibration. With exercise, however, capillary transit time may fall to the point that an alveolar-end capillary PO_2 difference develops, thereby worsening hypoxemia [1]. Modeling data suggest that at extremely high altitudes the pressure gradient may be small enough that an alveolar-end capillary PO_2 difference is seen even at rest [34].

In addition to the effects on gas diffusion, hypobaric hypoxia at high altitudes also alters ventilation–perfusion matching, particularly during exercise. This phenomenon was highlighted by Wagner et al. [35] who investigated the causes and effects of ventilation–perfusion inequality during a simulated ascent of Mount Everest. Their findings revealed that, at rest and with increasing physical exertion, ventilation–perfusion mismatch increased as barometric pressure decreased. The underlying causes of the increased inequality remain uncertain but may involve factors such as subclinical interstitial edema [36], uneven hypoxic pulmonary vasoconstriction leading to regional overperfusion [37], increased shunt through a patent foramen ovale present in approximately 30% of the population [38], or intrapulmonary arterio-venous anastomoses [39].

Lung Mechanics and Dynamics

In contrast to other aspects of respiratory system function, where the effects of hypobaric hypoxia are well-documented in terms of direction, magnitude, and timing, the changes in lung mechanics and dynamics after ascent to high altitude are less well understood. In part the unclear data result from small sample sizes in many studies and significant methodological differences between studies regarding the mode of hypoxia (simulated vs. terrestrial), the specific altitude studied, the timing of measurements after arrival, the rate of ascent, and the degree of physical activity among study participants.

Lung Mechanics Among the respiratory parameters studied under hypoxic conditions, vital capacity has shown the most consistent findings. Numerous studies investigating acute [40, 41] and subacute [42, 43] exposure to both natural high altitude [44] and simulated conditions [45] have reported reductions in vital capacity. The reasons for a reduced vital capacity remain unclear, though suggested mechanisms include interstitial fluid accumulation [43], reduced respiratory muscle strength [46], hypocapnia [47], and increased pulmonary blood volume [42]. However, relatively large and more recent studies [36, 48] found no significant changes in vital capacity within 2 days of ascent to 4559 m. Findings regarding static lung compliance are even less consistent, with studies reporting decreases [49], increases [50], or no changes [40] in this parameter at altitudes ranging from 3000 to 4559 m.

The observation that minute ventilation increases both at rest and during physical exertion at high altitudes raises questions about whether respiratory muscle strength and the capacity to maintain the increased work of breathing are affected. Research findings on respiratory muscle strength at rest have been inconsistent [46, 51, 52], while studies conducted during exercise indicate that various indicators of respiratory muscle performance, such as the diaphragm's force-generating capacity, time to exhaustion, and recovery time of the diaphragm, are impaired [53, 54]. The clinical significance of these changes, however, remains uncertain.

Lung Dynamics While certain factors at high altitudes, such as hypocapnia, increase airway resistance [55, 56], other factors like reduced air density and increased sympathetic nervous system activity during ascent [57] lower airway resistance. Because these factors simultaneously influence the airways during ascent to high altitude, it is not surprising that studies examining airway resistance at altitudes of 3400–5300 m have yielded mixed results, with some reporting decreased resistance [40, 44] or no change [48, 58]. Despite this variability, research consistently shows increased peak expiratory flow at high altitudes [46, 59], with the magnitude of this increase correlating with the altitude attained [43], likely due to a reduction in air density. Additionally, airway hyperresponsiveness is reduced at altitudes of 4559–5050 m in both healthy individuals [60] and those with well-controlled asthma [61].

Periodic Breathing

Even at elevations as low as 2500–3000 m, individuals often report disrupted sleep upon arrival at high altitude. These subjective experiences are linked to significant physiological alterations, including alterations in sleep architecture and episodes of periodic breathing, a form of central sleep apnea often seen at sea level in individuals with severe heart failure or various forms of neurologic injury.

Periodic breathing is characterized by a crescendo–decrescendo pattern of breathing movements and airflow, interrupted by periods of apnea lasting between

5 and 20 s. These apneas cause fluctuations in S_aO_2, with the lowest saturation level influenced by both the duration of apnea and the altitude at which one is sleeping. One factor contributing to the significant fluctuations in S_aO_2 with periodic breathing at high altitudes is that P_aO_2 typically falls on the steep portion of the hemoglobin–oxygen dissociation curve, where minor changes in P_aO_2 cause significant changes in S_aO_2 [11].

Periodic breathing commonly occurs during non-REM sleep and may even start during the drowsy state preceding sleep onset [62, 63]. Evidence suggests that when non-acclimatized lowlanders sleep at a constant elevation below 3000 m for several days, the duration of periodic breathing cycles generally decreases as the body acclimatizes, but increases at higher altitudes [1, 64]. For instance, several studies showed that when participants remained at a fixed altitude (ranging from 3450 to 5180 m) for 1–10 days, cycle length increased by 5–23% [65–68]. Similarly, in military recruits stationed at 4000 m, the average apnea duration extended from 12 s after 3 months to 16.5 s after 9 months [69]. While increasing S_pO_2 aligns with ventilatory acclimatization, it remains unclear if improved oxygen delivery directly contributes to the extension of cycle length. The observation that periodic breathing cycle length increases and persists, rather than diminishing with acclimatization, supports the idea that periodic breathing may serve as an adaptive response to high-altitude conditions, i.e., may represent a feature of VAH, rather than being a maladaptive effect [70]. However, in high-altitude-adapted highlanders, periodic breathing seems to be less pronounced compared to lowlanders [70]. These findings suggest that while periodic breathing continues to occur during high-altitude acclimatization without apparent negative effects, its significance diminishes with long-term adaptation to high altitude.

Periodic breathing has several effects beyond transient fluctuations in S_aO_2. Subjectively, individuals often report difficulty falling asleep or staying asleep, vivid dreams, frequent nighttime awakenings, and a feeling of not being refreshed upon awakening in the morning. Studies involving continuous electroencephalography (EEG) recordings, electromyography, and eye movement monitoring have identified an increased frequency of arousals [62, 71]. However, arousals at high altitude can also occur independently of periodic breathing [62, 72]. EEG studies have consistently shown changes in sleep architecture, including more time spent in lighter stages of non-REM sleep (stages I and II) and reduced time in deeper sleep stages [62, 73]. The impact on REM sleep is less clear, with some studies indicating a decrease [74] or even absence [75] of REM sleep, while others report no significant change [76] in the duration of this stage.

The mechanism underlying periodic breathing is complex and is best explained through the lens of control theory [77, 78]. A control system operates by initiating corrective actions in response to disturbances. An important factor in this context is an increased chemosensitivity to CO_2, both above and below normal levels of ventilation. This increased sensitivity causes excessive ventilatory responses to transient hypocapnia and to combined hypoxemic and hypercapnic chemoreceptor stimuli following apneas, sustaining the periodic breathing pattern [79, 80]. A strong ventilatory response to hypoxia can drive P_aCO_2 below the apnea threshold, which at high altitude during sleep lies only 1–2 mmHg below the eupneic P_aCO_2. When CO_2 chemosensitivity is high, the drop in P_aCO_2 triggers a cessation of ventilation. During the apnea, P_aCO_2 rises above the apnea threshold, eventually stimulating ventilation. Increased chemoreceptor sensitivity subsequently results in an excessive ventilatory response, causing P_aCO_2 to fall below the threshold once again, halting respiratory effort. This feedback loop produces an oscillatory pattern, where corrective adjustments in P_aCO_2 become misaligned with changes in ventilation, leading to amplification rather than stabilization.

Supplemental oxygen or oxygen-enriched sleeping environments can significantly reduce periodic breathing at high altitudes [81]. Additionally, medications such as the carbonic anhydrase inhibitor acetazolamide, and the phosphodiesterase inhibitor theophylline, reduce periodic breathing [82, 83], although the latter is not commonly used clinically due to its narrow therapeutic range. Sedative–hypnotic agents like zolpidem [84] and temazepam [85] improve subjective sleep quality at high altitude but have no measurable impact on periodic breathing.

Pulmonary Vascular Effects of Hypoxia

The impact of hypoxia on the pulmonary vasculature has been a subject of significant interest for more than 70 years. It is well established that alveolar hypoxia induces constriction of pulmonary arterioles, known as the von Euler–Liljestrand reflex or hypoxic pulmonary vasoconstriction (HPV) [86], thereby optimizing ventilation–perfusion matching and enhancing alveolar gas exchange by diverting blood flow from poorly ventilated to better-oxygenated areas of the lung. While localized HPV can be beneficial, as observed in conditions like pneumonia, widespread alveolar hypoxia at high altitudes triggers a more extensive and generalized HPV response, leading to increased pulmonary vascular resistance as all lung regions attempt unsuccessfully to divert blood flow elsewhere. At elevations >1600–2500 m [87, 88], along with a higher cardiac output, HPV increases pulmonary artery pressure and right ventricular afterload. However, the extent of HPV is not uniform across the lung and, similar to HVR, varies significantly (five-fold) among individuals [89]. Due to this regional variability, certain areas of the pulmonary vasculature with less HPV experience greater perfusion and higher downstream pressures than areas where arteriolar vasoconstriction is greater and the downstream vessels are under lesser pressure elevation. In individuals with an exaggerated HPV response, this uneven distribution of blood flow is considered to play a pivotal role in the development of high-altitude pulmonary edema (HAPE) [37, 90] as described below.

Hypoxic pulmonary vasoconstriction (HPV) occurs in multiple phases, with the initial response beginning almost immediately after exposure to hypoxia [91]. A second phase emerges approximately 2 h later, followed by a further rise in pulmonary artery pressure over the next 6–8 h [92]. The mechanisms driving HPV are intricate and primarily involve vascular smooth muscle in both the pulmonary arteries and veins. During the first phase, hypoxia stimulates the production of free radicals and reactive oxygen species, which increase intracellular Ca^{2+} concentration, leading to contraction of pulmonary vascular smooth muscle cells [93]. In the second phase, vasoconstriction is sustained due to a persistent reduction in nitric oxide bioavailability and an increase in vasoconstrictive factors such as endothelin-1 [94–96]. Various elements, including pulmonary innervation, circulating hormones, acid-base balance, and erythrocytes, influence these processes [97].

When hypoxia is brief (lasting hours to a few days), HPV can be fully reversed with supplemental oxygen [98]. However, prolonged exposure results in vascular remodeling, causing structural alterations in the pulmonary vasculature and reducing the reversibility of HPV with oxygen therapy [99–101]. This remodeling process is primarily driven by hypoxia-inducible factor (HIF) 1-α [102] and HIF 2-α [103], and involves excessive proliferation of endothelial cells, smooth muscle cells and fibroblasts, along with extracellular matrix deposition [104]. These changes contribute to vessel wall thickening and increased vascular stiffness. Although the exact timeline for remodeling and the reduced response to oxygen remains uncertain, it is believed to occur over days to weeks [98]. If persistent and untreated, the increased strain on the right ventricle can eventually lead to right heart failure in certain individuals [105].

High-Altitude Pulmonary Edema (HAPE)

HAPE is a pressure-induced, non-cardiac pulmonary edema that usually occurs within 1–5 days after an acute exposure to altitudes >3000 m when acclimatization is insufficient. Early symptoms include excessive dyspnea during exercise and reduced exercise performance. As edema progresses, orthopnea, gurgling in the chest, and pink frothy sputum occur. Under these circumstances, arterial oxygenation is significantly reduced, reflecting the severity of the disease. If untreated, the estimated mortality rate of HAPE is about 50% [106].

A key factor in the pathophysiology of HAPE is exaggerated HPV, leading to fluid leakage into the lungs. The critical role of a high pulmonary artery pressure is confirmed by the fact that descent, oxygen, or drugs that lower pulmonary artery pressure are effective for preventing and treating HAPE. Studies measuring plasma endothelin-1 [94], nitric oxide (NO) in exhaled air [107], NO metabolites in bronchoalveolar lavage fluid [108], and NO-dependent endothelial function in the systemic circulation [96] suggest that reduced NO availability and increased endothelin production under hypoxic conditions are the main factors underlying excessive HPV in HAPE-susceptible individuals. Additional mechanisms, e.g., inflammatory-induced increases in the permeability of the alveolar–capillary barrier and/or impaired alveolar fluid clearance, may contribute to the progression of HAPE following the initial hemodynamic pressure injury [108, 109].

The clearance of edema fluid from the alveolar space relies on the active transport of sodium (Na^+) and chloride (Cl^-) across alveolar epithelial type I and II cells

[110]. Na^+ enters these cells through various transporters on the apical membrane and is then expelled on the basolateral side via Na^+/K^+ pumps. Water follows passively, likely through paracellular pathways or aquaporins, which are water channels primarily located in alveolar epithelial type I cells. Once in the lung interstitium, the fluid is drained through the lymphatic system, which may be underdeveloped in individuals prone to HAPE [111]. It is well documented that hypoxia reduces transepithelial Na^+ transport (and thus alveolar fluid clearance) by decreasing the expression and activity of both epithelial Na^+ channels (ENaC) and the Na^+/K^+-ATPase. However, the extent to which impaired alveolar fluid clearance and lymphatic drainage contribute to HAPE pathophysiology remains unclear.

For preventing HAPE a gradual ascent profile is recommended. With travel >3000 m, individuals should not increase the sleeping elevation by more than 500 m/d and should include a rest day (i.e., no increase in sleeping elevation) every 3–4 days [112]. Pharmacologic prophylaxis should be considered for individuals with a history of HAPE. In such situations, nifedipine is the drug of choice [112] due to its pulmonary vasodilatory properties. If contraindications prohibit the intake of nifedipine, the phosphodiesterase-5-inhibitors tadalafil or sildenafil are recommended [112]. The carbonic anhydrase inhibitor acetazolamide is the mainstay of pharmacological prevention of acute mountain sickness, the most common acute high-altitude illness, but it is not recommended for preventing HAPE [112, 113]. Acetazolamide has been shown to be a potent inhibitor of acute HPV [114]. However, its ability to reduce hypoxic pulmonary artery pressure seems to decrease over time and it may not effectively attenuate HPV beyond 24 h [113].

In the treatment of HAPE, the most important measure is to reduce pulmonary vascular pressure and consequently the filtration of fluid into the lung. Oxygen counteracts HPV and should be started if available, followed by descent to a lower elevation. If descent is not feasible, supplemental oxygen should be continued or the individual should be placed in a portable hyperbaric chamber [112], which allows the exposure of a person to 105–165 mmHg above the ambient pressure by operating foot or hand driven pumps, thus simulating a descent of 1500–2500 m. Due to their pulmonary vasodilatory properties, nifedipine or phosphodiesterase-5-inhibitors (sildenafil or tadalafil) can serve as a supplementary treatment [112].

Conclusion

Each year, millions of individuals travel to high-altitude regions, and more than 80 million people reside permanently >2500 m. The reduced ambient PO_2 at these elevations initiates a series of physiological adaptations intended to maintain adequate oxygen supply at the tissue and cellular level. While the lung plays a central role in these adjustments, other organ systems (including the cardiovascular and the hematologic system, the kidneys, and the central nervous system) contribute significantly to maintaining oxygen delivery. Given adequate time for acclimatization, most individuals tolerate high-altitude hypoxia without difficulties. However, in some cases—particularly with excessively rapid ascent— maladaptive responses may arise, leading to acute high-altitude illness, the pulmonary manifestation of which is HAPE.

References

1. Berger MM, Luks AM. High altitude. Semin Respir Crit Care Med. 2023;44(5):681–95.
2. Clement ID, Bascom DA, Conway J, Dorrington KL, O'Connor DF, Painter R, et al. An assessment of central-peripheral ventilatory chemoreflex interaction in humans. Respir Physiol. 1992;88(1–2):87–100.
3. Clement ID, Pandit JJ, Bascom DA, Dorrington KL, O'Connor DF, Robbins PA. An assessment of central-peripheral ventilatory chemoreflex interaction using acid and bicarbonate infusions in humans. J Physiol. 1995;485(Pt 2):561–70.
4. Fatemian M, Nieuwenhuijs DJ, Teppema LJ, Meinesz S, van der Mey AG, Dahan A, et al. The respiratory response to carbon dioxide in humans with unilateral and bilateral resections of the carotid bodies. J Physiol. 2003;549(Pt 3):965–73.
5. Powell FL, Milsom WK, Mitchell GS. Time domains of the hypoxic ventilatory response. Respir Physiol. 1998;112(2):123–34.
6. Pamenter ME, Powell FL. Time domains of the hypoxic ventilatory response and their molecular basis. Compr Physiol. 2016;6(3):1345–85.
7. Vizek M, Pickett CK, Weil JV. Biphasic ventilatory response of adult cats to sustained hypoxia has central origin. J Appl Physiol (1985). 1987;63(4):1658–1664.
8. Ainslie PN, Lucas SJ, Burgess KR. Breathing and sleep at high altitude. Respir Physiol Neurobiol. 2013;188(3):233–56.
9. Teppema LJ, Dahan A. The ventilatory response to hypoxia in mammals: mechanisms, measurement, and analysis. Physiol Rev. 2010;90(2):675–754.
10. Rahn H, Otis AB. Man's respiratory response during and after acclimatization to high altitude. Am J Phys. 1949;157(3):445–62.
11. Luks AM, Ainslie PN, Lawley JS, Roach RC, Simonson TS. Ward, Milledge and West's high altitude medicine and physiology. Boca Raton: CRC Press; 2021. 544 p.
12. Wagner PD. Gas exchange. In: Hornbein TF, Schoene RB, editors. High altitude: an exploration of human adaptation. 161. New York: Marcel Dekker Inc; 2001. p. 199–234.
13. West JB. American medical research expedition to Everest. High Alt Med Biol. 2010;11(2):103–10.
14. West JB. Human physiology at extreme altitudes on Mount Everest. Science. 1984;223(4638):784–8.
15. Houston CS, Sutton JR, Cymerman A, Reeves JT. Operation Everest II: man at extreme altitude. J Appl Physiol. 1987;63(2):877–82.
16. Grocott MP, Martin DS, Levett DZ, McMorrow R, Windsor J, Montgomery HE. Arterial blood gases and oxygen content in climbers on Mount Everest. N Engl J Med. 2009;360(2):140–9.
17. Bernardi L, Schneider A, Pomidori L, Paolucci E, Cogo A. Hypoxic ventilatory response in successful extreme altitude climbers. Eur Respir J. 2006;27(1):165–71.
18. Meng L, Gelb AW. Regulation of cerebral autoregulation by carbon dioxide. Anesthesiology. 2015;122(1):196–205.
19. Oliveira DM, Rashid A, Brassard P, Silva BM. Exercise-induced potentiation of the acute hypoxic ventilatory response: neural mechanisms and implications for cerebral blood flow. Exp Physiol. 2024;109(11):1844–55.
20. Petrassi FA, Hodkinson PD, Walters PL, Gaydos SJ. Hypoxic hypoxia at moderate altitudes: review of the state of the science. Aviat Space Environ Med. 2012;83(10):975–84.

21. Sato M, Severinghaus JW, Powell FL, Xu FD, Spellman MJ Jr. Augmented hypoxic ventilatory response in men at altitude. J Appl Physiol (1985). 1992;73(1):101–7.
22. Forster HV, Dempsey JA, Birnbaum ML, Reddan WG, Thoden J, Grover RF, et al. Effect of chronic exposure to hypoxia on ventilatory response to CO_2 and hypoxia. J Appl Physiol. 1971;31(4):586–92.
23. Sorensen SC, Cruz JC. Ventilatory response to a single breath of CO_2 in O_2 in normal man at sea level and high altitude. J Appl Physiol. 1969;27(2):186–90.
24. Chiodi H. Respiratory adaptations to chronic high altitude hypoxia. J Appl Physiol. 1957;10(1):81–7.
25. West JB. Rate of ventilatory acclimatization to extreme altitude. Respir Physiol. 1988;74(3):323–33.
26. Burgess KR, Lucas SJ, Shepherd K, Dawson A, Swart M, Thomas KN, et al. Worsening of central sleep apnea at high altitude—a role for cerebrovascular function. J Appl Physiol (1985). 2013;114(8):1021–8.
27. Sato M, Severinghaus JW, Bickler P. Time course of augmentation and depression of hypoxic ventilatory responses at altitude. J Appl Physiol (1985). 1994;77(1):313–6.
28. Subudhi AW, Fan JL, Evero O, Bourdillon N, Kayser B, Julian CG, et al. AltitudeOmics: cerebral autoregulation during ascent, acclimatization, and re-exposure to high altitude and its relation with acute mountain sickness. J Appl Physiol (1985). 2014;116(7):724–729.
29. Tenney SM, Remmers JE, Mithoefer JC. Interaction of CO_2 and hypoxic stimuli on ventilation at high altitude. Q J Exp Physiol Cogn Med Sci. 1963;48:192–201.
30. Fan JL, Burgess KR, Thomas KN, Peebles KC, Lucas SJ, Lucas RA, et al. Influence of indomethacin on ventilatory and cerebrovascular responsiveness to CO_2 and breathing stability: the influence of PCO_2 gradients. Am J Physiol Regul Integr Comp Physiol. 2010;298(6):R1648–58.
31. Krapf R, Beeler I, Hertner D, Hulter HN, Chronic respiratory alkalosis. The effect of sustained hyperventilation on renal regulation of acid-base equilibrium. N Engl J Med. 1991;324(20):1394–401.
32. Schoene RB, Roach RC, Hackett PH, Sutton JR, Cymerman A, Houston CS. Operation Everest II: ventilatory adaptation during gradual decompression to extreme altitude. Med Sci Sports Exerc. 1990;22(6):804–10.
33. Piiper J, Scheid P. Model for capillary-alveolar equilibration with special reference to O_2 uptake in hypoxia. Respir Physiol. 1981;46(3):193–208.
34. West JB, Wagner PD. Predicted gas exchange on the summit of Mt. Everest. Respir Physiol. 1980;42(1):1–16.
35. Wagner PD, Sutton JR, Reeves JT, Cymerman A, Groves BM, Malconian MK. Operation Everest II: pulmonary gas exchange during a simulated ascent of Mt. Everest. J Appl Physiol. 1987;63(6):2348–59.
36. Cremona G, Asnaghi R, Baderna P, Brunetto A, Brutsaert T, Cavallaro C, et al. Pulmonary extravascular fluid accumulation in recreational climbers: a prospective study. Lancet. 2002;359(9303):303–9.
37. Dehnert C, Risse F, Ley S, Kuder TA, Buhmann R, Puderbach M, et al. Magnetic resonance imaging of uneven pulmonary perfusion in hypoxia in humans. Am J Respir Crit Care Med. 2006;174(10):1132–8.
38. Lovering AT, Kelly TS, DiMarco KG, Bradbury KE, Charkoudian N. Implications of a patent foramen ovale for environmental physiology and pathophysiology: do we know the 'hole' story? J Physiol. 2022;600(7):1541–53.
39. Lovering AT, Duke JW, Elliott JE. Intrapulmonary arteriovenous anastomoses in humans—response to exercise and the environment. J Physiol. 2015;593(3):507–20.
40. Gautier H, Peslin R, Grassino A, Milic-Emili J, Hannhart B, Powell E, et al. Mechanical properties of the lungs during acclimatization to altitude. J Appl Physiol Respir Environ Exerc Physiol. 1982;52(6):1407–15.

41. Senn O, Clarenbach CF, Fischler M, Thalmann R, Brunner-La Rocca H, Egger P, et al. Do changes in lung function predict high-altitude pulmonary edema at an early stage? Med Sci Sports Exerc. 2006;38(9):1565–70.
42. Welsh CH, Wagner PD, Reeves JT, Lynch D, Cink TM, Armstrong J, et al. Operation Everest. II: Spirometric and radiographic changes in acclimatized humans at simulated high altitudes. Am Rev Respir Dis. 1993;147(5):1239–44.
43. Mason NP, Barry PW, Pollard AJ, Collier DJ, Taub NA, Miller MR, et al. Serial changes in spirometry during an ascent to 5,300 m in the Nepalese Himalayas. High Alt Med Biol. 2000;1(3):185–95.
44. Mansell A, Powles A, Sutton J. Changes in pulmonary PV characteristics of human subjects at an altitude of 5,366 m. J Appl Physiol Respir Environ Exerc Physiol. 1980;49(1):79–83.
45. Finkelstein S, Tomashefski JF, Shillito FH. Pulmonary mechanics at altitude in normal and obstructive lung disease patients. Aerosp Med. 1965;36:880–4.
46. Deboeck G, Moraine JJ, Naeije R. Respiratory muscle strength may explain hypoxia-induced decrease in vital capacity. Med Sci Sports Exerc. 2005;37(5):754–8.
47. Swenson ER. Con: most climbers do not develop subclinical interstitial pulmonary edema. High Alt Med Biol. 2011;12(2):125–8; discussion 9–30.
48. Dehnert C, Luks AM, Schendler G, Menold E, Berger MM, Mairbaurl H, et al. No evidence for interstitial lung oedema by extensive pulmonary function testing at 4,559 m. Eur Respir J. 2010;35(4):812–20.
49. Jaeger JJ, Sylvester JT, Cymerman A, Berberich JJ, Denniston JC, Maher JT. Evidence for increased intrathoracic fluid volume in man at high altitude. J Appl Physiol. 1979;47(4):670–6.
50. Raymond L, Severinghaus JW. Static pulmonary compliance of man during altitude hypoxia. J Appl Physiol. 1971;31(5):785–7.
51. Forte VA Jr, Leith DE, Muza SR, Fulco CS, Cymerman A. Ventilatory capacities at sea level and high altitude. Aviat Space Environ Med. 1997;68(6):488–93.
52. Sharma S, Brown B. Spirometry and respiratory muscle function during ascent to higher altitudes. Lung. 2007;185(2):113–21.
53. Babcock MA, Johnson BD, Pegelow DF, Suman OE, Griffin D, Dempsey JA. Hypoxic effects on exercise-induced diaphragmatic fatigue in normal healthy humans. J Appl Physiol (1985). 1995;78(1):82–92.
54. Gudjonsdottir M, Appendini L, Baderna P, Purro A, Patessio A, Vilianis G, et al. Diaphragm fatigue during exercise at high altitude: the role of hypoxia and workload. Eur Respir J. 2001;17(4):674–80.
55. Newhouse MT, Becklake MR, Macklem PT, McGregor M. Effect of alterations in end-tidal CO_2 tension on flow resistance. J Appl Physiol. 1964;19:745–9.
56. van den Elshout FJ, van Herwaarden CL, Folgering HT. Effects of hypercapnia and hypocapnia on respiratory resistance in normal and asthmatic subjects. Thorax. 1991;46(1):28–32.
57. Mazzeo RS, Wolfel EE, Butterfield GE, Reeves JT. Sympathetic response during 21 days at high altitude (4,300 m) as determined by urinary and arterial catecholamines. Metabolism. 1994;43(10):1226–32.
58. Pellegrino R, Pompilio P, Quaranta M, Aliverti A, Kayser B, Miserocchi G, et al. Airway responses to methacholine and exercise at high altitude in healthy lowlanders. J Appl Physiol (1985). 2010;108(2):256–65.
59. Pollard AJ, Mason NP, Barry PW, Pollard RC, Collier DJ, Fraser RS, et al. Effect of altitude on spirometric parameters and the performance of peak flow meters. Thorax. 1996;51(2):175–8.
60. Pellegrino R, Viegi G, Brusasco V, Crapo RO, Burgos F, Casaburi R, et al. Interpretative strategies for lung function tests. Eur Respir J. 2005;26(5):948–68.
61. Cogo A, Basnyat B, Legnani D, Allegra L. Bronchial asthma and airway hyperresponsiveness at high altitude. Respiration. 1997;64(6):444–9.
62. Reite M, Jackson D, Cahoon RL, Weil JV. Sleep physiology at high altitude. Electroencephalogr Clin Neurophysiol. 1975;38(5):463–71.

63. Berssenbrugge A, Dempsey J, Iber C, Skatrud J, Wilson P. Mechanisms of hypoxia-induced periodic breathing during sleep in humans. J Physiol. 1983;343:507–24.
64. Bloch KE, Latshang TD, Turk AJ, Hess T, Hefti U, Merz TM, et al. Nocturnal periodic breathing during acclimatization at very high altitude at Mount Muztagh Ata (7,546 m). Am J Respir Crit Care Med. 2010;182(4):562–8.
65. Andrews G, Ainslie PN, Shepherd K, Dawson A, Swart M, Lucas S, et al. The effect of partial acclimatization to high altitude on loop gain and central sleep apnoea severity. Respirology. 2012;17(5):835–40.
66. Bird JD, Sands SA, Alex RM, Shing CLH, Shafer BM, Jendzjowsky NG, et al. Sex-related differences in loop gain during high-altitude sleep-disordered breathing. Ann Am Thorac Soc. 2023;20(8):1192–200.
67. Insalaco G, Romano S, Salvaggio A, Pomidori L, Mandolesi G, Cogo A. Periodic breathing, arterial oxyhemoglobin saturation, and heart rate during sleep at high altitude. High Alt Med Biol. 2012;13(4):258–62.
68. Kohler M, Kriemler S, Wilhelm EM, Brunner-LaRocca H, Zehnder M, Bloch KE. Children at high altitude have less nocturnal periodic breathing than adults. Eur Respir J. 2008;32(1):189–97.
69. Wang H, Li X, Li J, Gao Y, Li W, Zhao X, et al. Sleep, short-term memory, and mood states of volunteers with increasing altitude. Front Psych. 2022;13:952399.
70. Patrician A, Anholm JD, Ainslie PN. A narrative review of periodic breathing during sleep at high altitude: from acclimatizing lowlanders to adapted highlanders. J Physiol. 2024;602(21):5435–48.
71. Weil JV, Kryger MH, Scroggin CH. Sleep and breathing at high altitude. In: Guilleminault C, Dement WC, editors. Sleep apnea syndromes. New York: Alan R Liss; 1978. p. 119–23.
72. Wickramasinghe H, Anholm JD. Sleep and breathing at high altitude. Sleep Breath. 1999;3(3):89–102.
73. Joern AT, Shurley JT, Brooks RE, Guenter CA, Pierce CM. Short-term changes in sleep patterns on arrival at the South Polar Plateau. Arch Intern Med. 1970;125(4):649–54.
74. Anholm JD, Powles AC, Downey R 3rd, Houston CS, Sutton JR, Bonnet MH, et al. Operation Everest II: arterial oxygen saturation and sleep at extreme simulated altitude. Am Rev Respir Dis. 1992;145(4 Pt 1):817–26.
75. Pappenheimer JR. Sleep and respiration of rats during hypoxia. J Physiol. 1977;266(1):191–207.
76. Zielinski J, Koziej M, Mankowski M, Sarybaev AS, Tursalieva JS, Sabirov IS, et al. The quality of sleep and periodic breathing in healthy subjects at an altitude of 3,200 m. High Alt Med Biol. 2000;1(4):331–6.
77. Cherniack NS, Longobardo GS. Mathematical models of periodic breathing and their usefulness in understanding cardiovascular and respiratory disorders. Exp Physiol. 2006;91(2):295–305.
78. Khoo MC, Kronauer RE, Strohl KP, Slutsky AS. Factors inducing periodic breathing in humans: a general model. J Appl Physiol Respir Environ Exerc Physiol. 1982;53(3):644–59.
79. Dempsey JA. Crossing the apnoeic threshold: causes and consequences. Exp Physiol. 2005;90(1):13–24.
80. Khoo MC. Determinants of ventilatory instability and variability. Respir Physiol. 2000;122(2–3):167–82.
81. Lahiri S, Maret K, Sherpa MG. Dependence of high altitude sleep apnea on ventilatory sensitivity to hypoxia. Respir Physiol. 1983;52(3):281–301.
82. Hackett PH, Roach RC, Harrison GL, Schoene RB, Mills WJ Jr. Respiratory stimulants and sleep periodic breathing at high altitude. Almitrine versus acetazolamide. Am Rev Respir Dis. 1987;135(4):896–8.
83. Fischer R, Lang SM, Leitl M, Thiere M, Steiner U, Huber RM. Theophylline and acetazolamide reduce sleep-disordered breathing at high altitude. Eur Respir J. 2004;23(1):47–52.

84. Beaumont M, Goldenberg F, Lejeune D, Marotte H, Harf A, Lofaso F. Effect of zolpidem on sleep and ventilatory patterns at simulated altitude of 4,000 meters. Am J Respir Crit Care Med. 1996;153(6 Pt 1):1864–9.
85. Nickol AH, Leverment J, Richards P, Seal P, Harris GA, Cleland J, et al. Temazepam at high altitude reduces periodic breathing without impairing next-day performance: a randomized cross-over double-blind study. J Sleep Res. 2006;15(4):445–54.
86. von Euler US, Liljestrand G. Observations on the pulmonary arterial blood pressure in the cat. Acta Physiol Scand. 1946;12:301–20.
87. Levine BD, Zuckerman JH, deFilippi CR. Effect of high-altitude exposure in the elderly: the Tenth Mountain Division study. Circulation. 1997;96(4):1224–32.
88. Swenson ER, Robertson HT, Hlastala MP. Effects of inspired carbon dioxide on ventilation-perfusion matching in normoxia, hypoxia, and hyperoxia. Am J Respir Crit Care Med. 1994;149(6):1563–9.
89. Grunig E, Mereles D, Hildebrandt W, Swenson ER, Kubler W, Kuecherer H, et al. Stress Doppler echocardiography for identification of susceptibility to high altitude pulmonary edema. J Am Coll Cardiol. 2000;35(4):980–7.
90. Hopkins SR, Garg J, Bolar DS, Balouch J, Levin DL. Pulmonary blood flow heterogeneity during hypoxia and high-altitude pulmonary edema. Am J Respir Crit Care Med. 2005;171(1):83–7.
91. Talbot NP, Balanos GM, Dorrington KL, Robbins PA. Two temporal components within the human pulmonary vascular response to approximately 2 h of isocapnic hypoxia. J Appl Physiol (1985). 2005;98(3):1125–39.
92. Vejlstrup NG, O'Neill M, Nagyova B, Dorrington KL. Time course of hypoxic pulmonary vasoconstriction: a rabbit model of regional hypoxia. Am J Respir Crit Care Med. 1997;155(1):216–21.
93. Smith KA, Schumacker PT. Sensors and signals: the role of reactive oxygen species in hypoxic pulmonary vasoconstriction. J Physiol. 2019;597(4):1033–43.
94. Berger MM, Dehnert C, Bailey DM, Luks AM, Menold E, Castell C, et al. Transpulmonary plasma ET-1 and nitrite differences in high altitude pulmonary hypertension. High Alt Med Biol. 2009;10(1):17–24.
95. Bailey DM, Dehnert C, Luks AM, Menold E, Castell C, Schendler G, et al. High-altitude pulmonary hypertension is associated with a free radical-mediated reduction in pulmonary nitric oxide bioavailability. J Physiol. 2010;588(Pt 23):4837–47.
96. Berger MM, Hesse C, Dehnert C, Siedler H, Kleinbongard P, Bardenheuer HJ, et al. Hypoxia impairs systemic endothelial function in individuals prone to high-altitude pulmonary edema. Am J Respir Crit Care Med. 2005;172(6):763–7.
97. Swenson ER. Hypoxic pulmonary vasoconstriction. High Alt Med Biol. 2013;14(2):101–10.
98. Subedi P, Gasho C, Stembridge M, Williams AM, Patrician A, Ainslie PN, et al. Pulmonary vascular reactivity to supplemental oxygen in Sherpa and lowlanders during gradual ascent to high altitude. Exp Physiol. 2023;108(1):111–22.
99. Berger MM, Bailey DM. On the mechanisms underlying activation and reversal of high altitude-induced pulmonary hypertension in humans—another piece in the pulmonary puzzle. Exp Physiol. 2023;108(1):1–4.
100. Sylvester JT, Shimoda LA, Aaronson PI, Ward JP. Hypoxic pulmonary vasoconstriction. Physiol Rev. 2012;92(1):367–520.
101. Luks AM, Levett D, Martin DS, Goss CH, Mitchell K, Fernandez BO, et al. Changes in acute pulmonary vascular responsiveness to hypoxia during a progressive ascent to high altitude (5300 m). Exp Physiol. 2017;102(6):711–24.
102. Pugh CW. Modulation of the hypoxic response. Adv Exp Med Biol. 2016;903:259–71.
103. Slingo ME. Oxygen-sensing pathways and the pulmonary circulation. J Physiol. 2024;602(21):5619–29.
104. Shimoda LA. Cellular pathways promoting pulmonary vascular remodeling by hypoxia. Physiology (Bethesda). 2020;35(4):222–33.

105. Sydykov A, Mamazhakypov A, Maripov A, Kosanovic D, Weissmann N, Ghofrani HA, et al. Pulmonary hypertension in acute and chronic high altitude maladaptation disorders. Int J Environ Res Public Health. 2021;18(4)
106. Bartsch P, Swenson ER. Clinical practice: acute high-altitude illnesses. N Engl J Med. 2013;368(24):2294–302.
107. Busch T, Bartsch P, Pappert D, Grunig E, Hildebrandt W, Elser H, et al. Hypoxia decreases exhaled nitric oxide in mountaineers susceptible to high-altitude pulmonary edema. Am J Respir Crit Care Med. 2001;163(2):368–73.
108. Swenson ER, Maggiorini M, Mongovin S, Gibbs JS, Greve I, Mairbaurl H, et al. Pathogenesis of high-altitude pulmonary edema: inflammation is not an etiologic factor. JAMA. 2002;287(17):2228–35.
109. Sartori C, Allemann Y, Duplain H, Lepori M, Egli M, Lipp E, et al. Salmeterol for the prevention of high-altitude pulmonary edema. N Engl J Med. 2002;346(21):1631–6.
110. Matthay MA, Clerici C, Saumon G. Invited review: active fluid clearance from the distal air spaces of the lung. J Appl Physiol. 2002;93(4):1533–41.
111. Carter EA, Mayo JR, MacInnis MJ, McKenzie DC, Koehle MS. Individual susceptibility to high altitude and immersion pulmonary edema and pulmonary lymphatics. Aviat Space Environ Med. 2014;85(1):9–14.
112. Luks AM, Beidleman BA, Freer L, Grissom CK, Keyes LE, McIntosh SE, et al. Wilderness Medical Society clinical practice guidelines for the prevention, diagnosis, and treatment of acute altitude illness: 2024 update. Wilderness Environ Med. 2024;35(1_suppl):2S–19S.
113. Berger MM, Sareban M, Schiefer LM, Swenson KE, Treff F, Schafer L, et al. Effects of acetazolamide on pulmonary artery pressure and prevention of high-altitude pulmonary edema after rapid active ascent to 4,559 m. J Appl Physiol (1985). 2022;132(6):1361–9.
114. Boulet LM, Teppema LJ, Hackett HK, Dominelli PB, Cheyne WS, Dominelli GS, et al. Attenuation of human hypoxic pulmonary vasoconstriction by acetazolamide and methazolamide. J Appl Physiol (1985). 2018;125:1795–803.
115. Sareban M, Schiefer LM, Macholz F, Schafer L, Zangl Q, Inama F, et al. Endurance athletes are at increased risk for early acute mountain sickness at 3450 m. Med Sci Sports Exerc. 2019;52:1109.
116. Berger MM, Macholz F, Lehmann L, Dankl D, Hochreiter M, Bacher B, et al. Remote ischemic preconditioning does not prevent acute mountain sickness after rapid ascent to 3,450 m. J Appl Physiol (1985). 2017;123(5):1228–34.
117. Berger MM, Macholz F, Sareban M, Schmidt P, Fried S, Dankl D, et al. Inhaled budesonide does not prevent acute mountain sickness after rapid ascent to 4559 m. Eur Respir J. 2017;50(3):pii: 1700982.
118. Smith TG, Dempsey JA, Hornbein TF. Control of breathing at high altitude. In: Hornbein TF, Schoene RB, editors. High altitude: an exploration of human adaptation (Lung biology in health and disease). 161. New York: Marcel Dekker; 2001. p. 140–8.

Chapter 4
Breathing in Space

Jan Stepanek, Dakota McNierney, and Wiaam Elkhatib

Introduction

The striking increase in governmental and private human space flight activity with flights to suborbital, orbital, lunar, and eventually planned Mars destinations is raising the importance of clinicians' understanding of adaptive changes that occur during space flight activities, as well as clinical risks contingent on the duration and nature of the planned activity. The purpose of this review is to provide clinicians with a framework to categorize changes and specific risks while they care for either healthy participants or individuals with preexisting pulmonary conditions engaged in space flight. This chapter will not address off-nominal operational emergency scenarios, such as fire, accidents, or accidental decompressions.

J. Stepanek (✉)
Aerospace Medicine Program, Department of Medicine, Mayo Clinic, Phoenix, AZ, USA
e-mail: stepanek.jan@mayo.edu

D. McNierney
Division of Pulmonary and Sleep Medicine, Department of Medicine, Mayo Clinic, Phoenix, AZ, USA

Department of Critical Care Medicine, Mayo Clinic, Phoenix, AZ, USA
e-mail: mcnierney.dakota@mayo.edu

W. Elkhatib
Division of Public Health, Infectious Disease and Occupational Medicine; Aerospace Medicine, Mayo Clinic, Rochester, MN, USA
e-mail: elkhatib.wiaam@mayo.edu

E. R. Swenson, A. M. Luks (eds.), *The Lungs at the Extremes of Environment and Age*, Respiratory Medicine, https://doi.org/10.1007/978-3-031-98371-9_4

Terminology

Suborbital spaceflight is a term applied to flights that attain an altitude of greater than or equal to 100 km (Karman line), lasting no more than several hours, depending on the specific space vehicle and mission, with brief exposure to increased gravity and several minutes of microgravity.

Orbital flights typically occur in low Earth orbit (<2000 km) with destinations such as the International Space Station (ISS) at an altitude of 340 km above Earth. Contingent on the mission profile, these flights can last days to months with prolonged exposure to microgravity and increased gravity exposure upon launch and reentry.

Lunar flights are expected to last from weeks to months, depending on the mission profile, with exposure to increased gravity upon launch, prolonged exposure to microgravity during the journey to the Moon, and, on the Moon's surface, exposure to reduced gravity of 1.6 m/s^2.

Mars missions will last months to years, contingent on the mission profile and planned activities. Extended-duration exposure to microgravity, as well as transient increases in gravity during launch and landing, are expected, as well as exposure to a gravitational force of 3.7 m/s^2 on the surface of Mars (terrestrial gravity is by comparison at 9.81 m/s^2).

Physiology

Gas Laws

The application of the gas laws provides a sound understanding of the physiological challenges that space flight imposes on the human respiratory system.

Boyle's Law Boyle's law states that at a constant temperature, the pressure and volume of a gas are inversely proportional.

$$P_1 \times V_1 = P_2 \times V_2 \tag{4.1}$$

where P_1 = first pressure, P_2 = second pressure, V_1 = first volume, and V_2 = second volume.

For a wet gas, the relationship is expressed as:

$$\left(P_1 - P_{H_2O}\right) \times V_1 = \left(P_2 - P_{P_{H_2O}}\right) \times V_2 \tag{4.2}$$

where P_{H_2O} refers to water vapor pressure.

The Earth's atmospheric pressure at sea level is 760 mmHg or 1 atmosphere (atm), which is equivalent to 1013.25 millibars or 14.7 pounds per square inch. It comprises a layer of gases, primarily composed of nitrogen (79%) and oxygen

(20.9%). During inspiration, the diaphragm and external intercostal muscles contract, causing the thoracic cavity to expand, resulting in an increase in lung volume. This creates a pressure gradient with lower pressure within the lungs than the atmosphere, resulting in air flowing from the environment into the lungs. Note the importance of taking into account the effect of water vapor for biological systems that are water saturated, as larger volume expansion occurs upon decreases in pressure [1]. In space, barometric pressure is absent, which means that any gas in the body will increase its volume. The space vehicle and spacesuit must control the pressure around the human body to ensure that gases within the body do not expand rapidly and cause decompression sickness (DCS) and illness.

Henry's Law Henry's law also has several important implications in spaceflight. It states that the amount of gas dissolved in a liquid is directly proportional to the partial pressure of the gas above (i.e., in equilibrium with) the liquid at a constant temperature.

$$\text{Henry's Law}: C = \text{KP} \times P \quad (4.3)$$

where C = concentration of the gas in the liquid, KP = Henry's law constant for that gas in the liquid, and P = partial pressure of the gas above the liquid.

The vacuum of space has a significant effect on dissolved gases in a biological system. With a sudden reduction in external pressure, gas will no longer remain dissolved in liquids, such as bodily fluids, and instead will come out of solution in the gas phase. This can lead to the formation of nitrogen bubbles in the bloodstream and tissues, a phenomenon known as decompression sickness (DCS), often referred to as "the bends." This problem could develop, for example, if a spacecraft malfunctions and depressurizes [1].

Dalton's Law Dalton's law of partial pressures becomes relevant when reviewing how each individual gas is impacted in space. The law states that in a mixture of nonreacting gases, the total pressure of the gas exerted is equal to the sum of the partial pressures of the individual gases.

$$P_{\text{total}} = P_1 + P_2 + P_3 + \cdots \quad (4.4)$$

where P_1, P_2, P_3,… are the partial pressures of constituent gases.

As altitude increases, atmospheric pressure decreases, and the partial pressure of each individual gas also decreases. The partial pressure of a gas is responsible for the physiological effects of that gas. This becomes crucial for oxygenation, as these gases follow a pressure gradient, moving from an area of high partial pressure to an area of low partial pressure. At 1 atm, the partial pressure of oxygen is higher in the air and alveoli than in the bloodstream, leading to diffusion of oxygen into the bloodstream. In space, there is no atmospheric pressure; therefore, upon exposure to the vacuum of space, the flux of gas would be from the human body into the ambient vacuum resulting in severe, lethal hypoxemia [1]. This is why a carefully controlled environment such as a spacecraft or spacesuit is critical for satisfactory physiologic function and survival.

Respiratory Mechanics

The respiratory system allows us to extract oxygen from the environment and expel carbon dioxide, maintaining acid-base homeostasis. The mechanics of breathing rely on the interaction between lung compliance, chest wall compliance, respiratory rate, and airway resistance to create pressure gradients within the lungs and thoracic cavity [2]. This process is facilitated by the diaphragm and intercostal muscles and is affected by gravity, contingent on body position on Earth. Inhalation occurs when the diaphragm contracts (alongside contributions from external intercostal muscles), causing it to flatten and move downward, increasing the volume of the thoracic cavity [2]. As the thoracic cavity's volume increases, the pressure in the pleural space and airspaces decreases, creating a pressure gradient which allows inward movement of air. Once the pressure at the mouth and alveolar pressure come into equilibrium, inhalation stops. As the diaphragm relaxes, the elastic recoil of the lungs increases alveolar pressure above the pressure at the mouth, setting up a pressure gradient for expiratory flow, which facilitates the elimination of carbon dioxide.

Ventilation/Perfusion

For efficient gas exchange between the alveoli and capillaries, each alveolus must be adequately ventilated and perfused. Ventilation ($\dot{V}_A$) refers to the flow of air into the alveoli, as described above, while perfusion ($\dot{Q}$) is the blood flow to the alveolar capillaries. The adequacy of ventilation–perfusion matching is assessed using the ventilation to perfusion ratio ($\dot{V}_A/\dot{Q}$). In an ideal lung, the $\dot{V}_A/\dot{Q}$ ratio should be 1, indicating that the ventilation and perfusion are well matched. However, the ratio varies throughout the lung as ventilation and blood flow are unevenly distributed due to airway and vascular tree geometries and the influence of gravity on hydrostatic pressures. The relationship between alveolar pressure, arterial pressure, and venous pressure varies depending on the region of the lung examined, as conceptualized in the West zones of pulmonary perfusion. This model postulates that there is a vertical gradient of perfusion within the lungs directly influenced by gravity. These regions were divided into three zones. Zone 1 is the area toward the apex of the lung where alveolar pressure is higher than both arterial and venous pressures such that alveolar units receive ventilation but no perfusion. Zone 2 is defined as the area of the lung where the alveolar pressure is higher than venous pressure such that the driving pressure for blood flow is now the difference between arterial and alveolar pressure. Zone 3 is the area where both arterial and venous pressures are higher than alveolar pressure such that the driving pressure for blood flow is now the

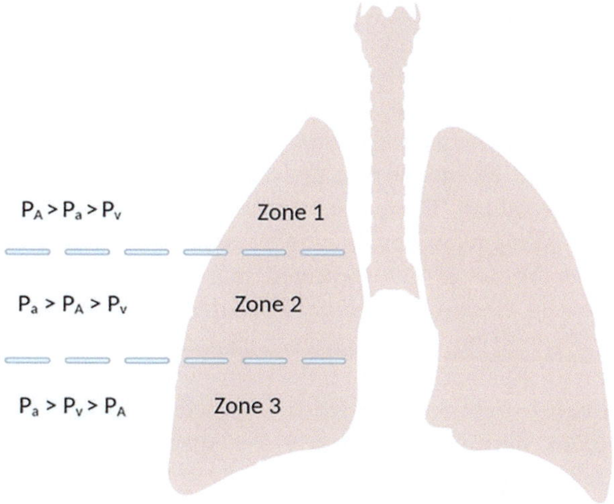

Fig. 4.1 Diagram illustrating the zonal perfusion patterns of the upright lung (P_a pulmonary arterial pressure, P_A pulmonary alveolar pressure, P_v pulmonary venous pressure). (Created in BioRender. McNierney, D. (2025) https://BioRender.com/4r47hes)

difference between arterial and venous pressure. This driving pressure is higher than in Zone 2 with the net result being that alveolar units in Zone 3 receive more blood flow (Fig. 4.1).

In the upright position, gravity increases blood flow to the dependent (i.e., lower) portions of the lung. This results, on average, in a five-fold lower $\dot{V}_A/\dot{Q}$ ratio in the base compared to the apex of the lung [3]. Any significant changes in ventilation or perfusion can impact this ratio, leading to alterations in gas exchange, resulting in possible hypoxemia.

In microgravity, both ventilation and perfusion are more uniformly distributed, reducing physiological dead space and recruiting more vasculature to participate in gas exchange [4]. Despite the greater uniformity of ventilation–perfusion matching, areas of inhomogeneity persist. This highlights the spatial interdependence of ventilation and perfusion, as the airways and vasculature have fixed anatomical relationships (fractal geometry), with airways and pulmonary arteries branching in union with each other [4, 5]. Regardless of the absence of gravity, regional ventilation and perfusion are matched and remain comparable to values seen at 1 atm [6].

Lung Volumes

Pulmonary function testing allows for measurement of lung volumes and lung capacities during inspiration and expiration. The functional residual capacity (FRC) is the volume of gas present in the lung at the end of tidal exhalation [6]. This value represents the point where alveolar pressure is the same as the pressure at the mouth (i.e., atmospheric pressure). As mentioned above, gravity plays an important role in ventilation and is impacted by body position. A systematic review of 43 studies, for example, revealed that forced expiratory volume in one second (FEV_1), forced vital capacity (FVC), and FRC to be higher in an upright position compared to supine position on Earth [7].

Edyvean et al. studied the effect of 15–20 s of microgravity on the lungs, chest wall, and abdominal compartment [8] and found a 244 mL decrease in FRC, a 63% increase in abdominal compliance, a 225 mL increase in rib cage compartment volume, and an increase in the diaphragm–abdominal compartment contribution to tidal breathing. These results were attributed to the effect of gravitational unloading of the diaphragm, resulting in a cranial shift of the diaphragm–abdominal compartment. These results indicated that 0G respiratory mechanics are intermediate between those in the upright and supine postures at 1G.

The first study that examined alterations in lung volumes during sustained microgravity was performed in 1991 during the Spacelab Life Sciences-1 (SLS-1) mission [9]. Pulmonary function tests were performed (Fig. 4.3) on four individuals before, during, and after a 9-day Spacelab SLS-1 shuttle mission. Compared to preflight measurements, FRC fell by 15% (500 mL) in microgravity and by 32% in the supine position on Earth, while expiratory reserve volume (ERV) was reduced by 10–20% in microgravity and by 64% in the supine position on Earth. Residual volume (RV) was reduced by 18% (310 mL) in microgravity but did not significantly change in the supine position on Earth. Tidal volume (V_T) decreased by 15% in microgravity (90 mL), but the supine V_T was unchanged compared with preflight standing values. Total lung capacity (TLC) decreased by 8% during microgravity and in the supine position on Earth when compared with preflight standing values. Vital capacity (VC) was reduced by around 10% after 24 h in microgravity; however, after 4–9 days in microgravity, it returned to its preflight value. The reductions in FRC, ERV, and RV during microgravity were attributed to the cranial shift of the diaphragm, increased intrathoracic blood volume, and more uniform alveolar expansion [9] (Fig. 4.2).

These studies show that in a microgravity environment, ERV is significantly reduced, VC is unaltered after initial decline, and FRC is intermediate between that in the upright and supine position at 1G (Fig. 4.3).

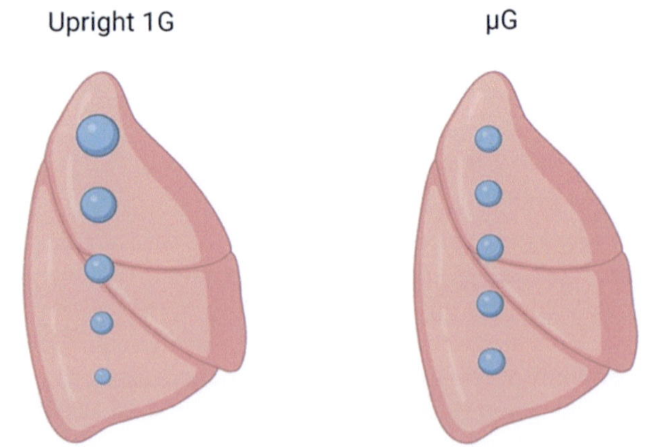

Fig. 4.2 Illustration of alveolar volume changes in terrestrial gravity (1G) and microgravity (μG) environments. (Created in BioRender. McNierney, D. (2025) https://BioRender.com/a75e768)

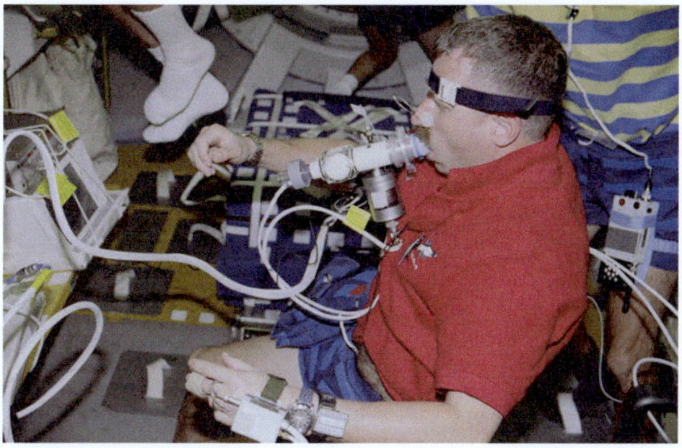

Fig. 4.3 Astronaut David Williams is pictured during a Neurolab pulmonary function test. Williams joined four NASA astronauts and two payload specialists for 16 days aboard the Space Shuttle Columbia in support of the Neurolab mission. (Photo credit: NASA)

Diffusing Capacity

The diffusing capacity for carbon monoxide (D_LCO) is a measure of the ability to transfer gases from the alveoli into the bloodstream [10]. Fick's law of diffusion describes the process of gas exchange across the alveolar–capillary barrier.

$$(J) = \left[(A \cdot D \cdot \Delta P) / T \right] \quad (4.5)$$

where J = rate of diffusion, A = surface area of the membrane through which diffusion occurs, D = diffusion coefficient of the gas, ΔP = difference in partial pressure of the gas across the membrane, and T = thickness of the membrane.

This relationship demonstrates how different factors influence the diffusion of gases in the lungs. The diffusion coefficient is influenced by molecular size, temperature, alveolar membrane properties, and gas density, while the partial pressure gradient is determined by the alveolar gas mixture, the partial pressure of the gas and gas concentration. The alveolar–capillary membrane thickness and surface area, as well as capillary transit time and protein-gas binding, also play a significant role.

In microgravity, D_LCO increases significantly, remains at that level throughout the microgravity exposure, and returns to preflight values immediately upon re-entry to 1G [11–13]. Prisk et al., for example, found that diffusing capacity increased by 18% when compared to 1G standing values but was not significantly different from 1G supine values and remained constant throughout the 9-day flight. This is likely due to more uniform capillary filling in the nondependent areas of the lungs in the absence of gravity, which serves to increase the surface area of the interface between the alveoli and capillaries (A in Fick's Law) [14].

Cardiopulmonary Interaction

When a person is in the upright position in the 1G gravity environment of Earth, gravity causes blood to pool in the lower extremities. The venous system has thinner, less muscular, and more distensible walls, which allow it to function as capacitance vessels capable of accommodating hydrostatic volume shifts. This increase in venous volume and pressure in the lower extremities decreases thoracic venous volume and central venous pressure (CVP), which, in turn, reduces preload and, in accordance with the Frank–Starling mechanism, limits stroke volume. The intricate design of the human body has regulatory mechanisms to compensate for the decreased arterial pressure. Baroreceptors in the aortic arch and carotid arteries are activated to restore normal arterial pressure, primarily through systemic vasoconstriction and increased sympathoadrenal tone (positive inotrope and chronotropic effects) [13] (Fig. 4.4).

In a microgravity environment, the gravitational influence on the pulmonary and cardiovascular system is removed, causing an immediate shift of fluid to the central compartment [14]. This central fluid shift dilates the central vasculature and increases cardiac output by up to 18% after 24 h of microgravity exposure [15] (Fig. 4.5). It was previously hypothesized that increased thoracic venous volume

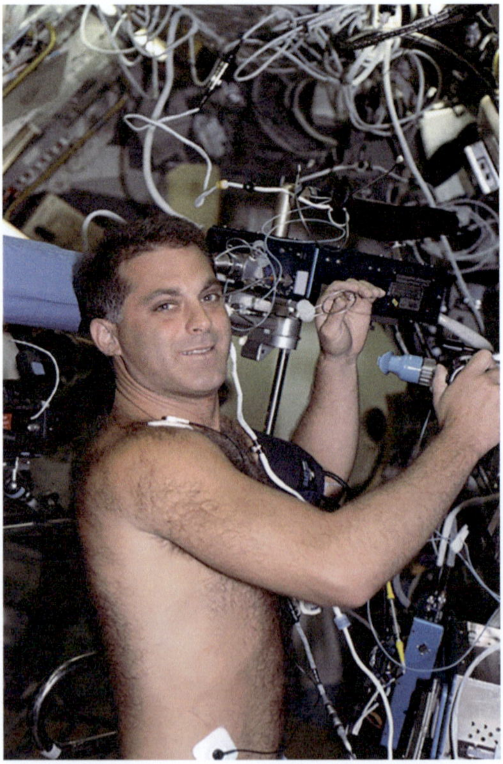

Fig. 4.4 Astronaut David A. Wolf is completing a test that investigates the in-space distribution and movement of blood and gas in the pulmonary system during the STS-58 mission. The results were then compared to testing performed on Earth to determine the changes that occur in pulmonary function in space. (Photo credit: NASA)

would increase CVP; however, it has been found that CVP declines in microgravity. Buckey et al. [16] found that even with the fall in CVP, the left ventricular end-diastolic dimension measured by echocardiography increased within 48 h, indicating that the relationship between CVP and transmural left ventricular pressures is altered in microgravity. An explanation for this phenomenon is that once gravity is removed, chest cavity volume increases, resulting in intrapleural pressures becoming more negative. This increases right ventricular preload, which, in turn, increases cardiac transmural pressure and, despite the fluid shift, decreases CVP. This concept was further supported by Videbaek et al. who concluded that during short periods of microgravity, CVP and esophageal pressures decreased while left atrial diameter increased [17].

Effects of G*-Forces*

When a spacecraft fires its propulsion system to escape Earth's gravity and then reenters the atmosphere, the resulting forces (*G*-forces) have significant physiologic consequences contingent on the direction of the forces acting upon the human body (Fig. 4.5). Most space-vehicle systems orient the occupants in $+G_x$ position (inertial force acting chest-to-back) to minimize negative impacts on cerebral perfusion, as

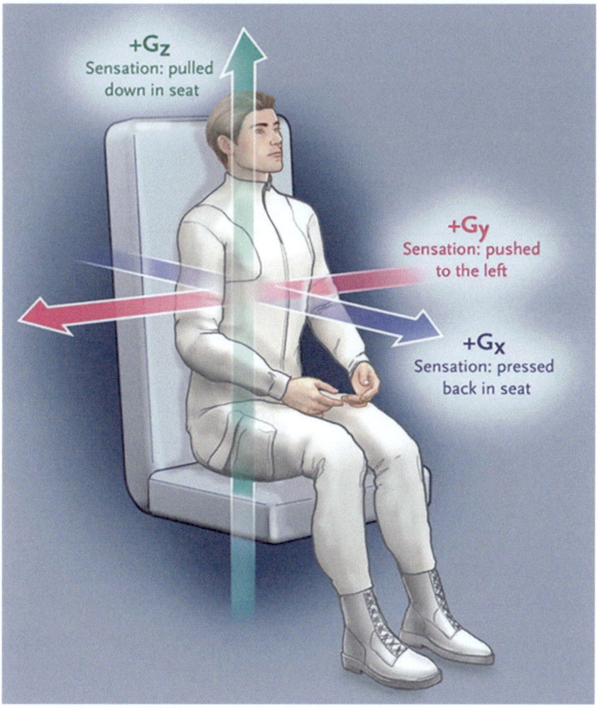

Fig. 4.5 Acceleration vectors and associated inertial force sensations. (© The *New England Journal of Medicine* (2025))

would be expected with inertial forces acting in head-to-toe acceleration direction ($+G_z$). In healthy subjects, the increased work of breathing, increased respiratory rate, decreased vital capacity, increased ventilation–perfusion mismatch, and mild resultant hypoxemia with increasing $+G_x$ may result in symptoms consistent with symptomatic respiratory alkalosis secondary to increased ventilation [18]. While the time periods of *G*-exposure are brief and generally well-tolerated in young, healthy cohorts based on centrifuge studies, they pose a risk of respiratory impairment in those with underlying pulmonary disease, neuromuscular or diaphragmatic function disorders, obesity, or poor fitness. Such interactions are highly individualized and require medical assessment in collaboration with the spaceflight medical team.

The effects of acceleration on pulmonary function during the flight phases of increased gravitational forces have been demonstrated in terrestrial models of human cardiorespiratory physiology, such as human centrifuges or data gathered during high-performance flight. Acceleration back to front ($+G_x$ inertial forces) is the most important cause of physiologic alterations [19]. The inertial forces acting upon an occupant increase ventilation–perfusion mismatch, due to increased perfusion and reduced ventilation in posterior lung tissues, thereby increasing the shunt fraction and causing hypoxemia.

Lung mechanics are also altered. A decrease in vital capacity is evident (50% decrease at $+6G_x$) and accompanied by a marked reduction in expiratory reserve volume, and work of breathing increases with increased $+G_x$ forces [19]. Residual volume appears to be preserved, though functional residual capacity is overly sensitive to acceleration forces as it is based on mere body posture.

The astronaut or high-performance pilot is typically provided a high inspired oxygen fraction (F_IO_2) during the critical phases of take-off and landing while in their suits. The combination of increased gravitational inertial forces (typically $+G_x$) and the use of high F_IO_2 increases the risk that some lung regions become atelectatic, which further worsens gas exchange [18, 20] (Fig. 4.6).

Threats

Pulmonary Barotrauma

As atmospheric pressure decreases, any trapped air within the lungs will expand and potentially lead to pneumothorax, pneumomediastinum, hemorrhage [21], or arterial or venous gas embolization. This risk must be considered in any candidate for space flight with underlying pulmonary disease associated with airflow obstruction or bullae and cyst formation, such as individuals with asthma, chronic obstructive pulmonary disease, bullous emphysema, or cystic fibrosis. Preflight testing should be considered in such individuals including evaluation of suspected trapped gas volume in the lung with imaging and gas washout methods contingent on the

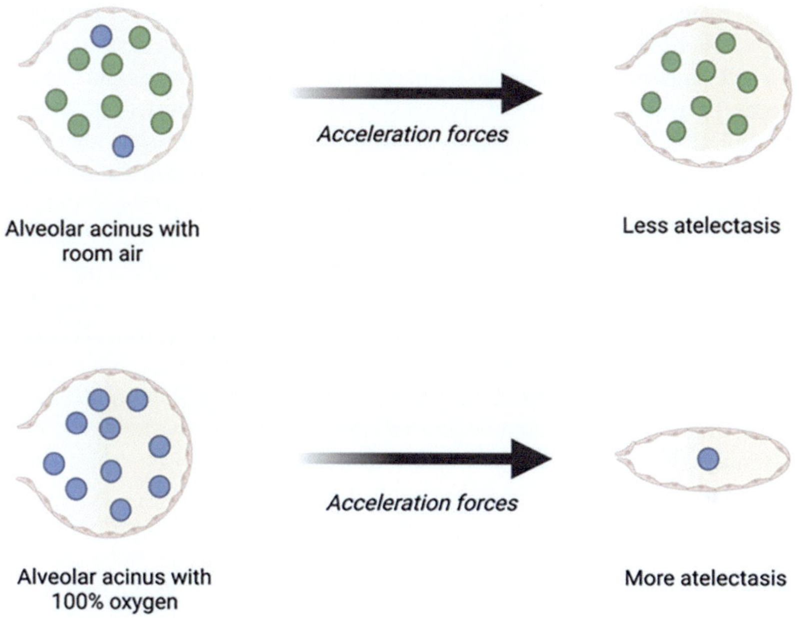

Fig. 4.6 Lung tissue atelectasis propensity under acceleration forces is contingent on the composition of inhaled gas (blue: absorbable oxygen; green: inert nitrogen). (Created in BioRender. Stepanek, J. (2025) https://BioRender.com/4spws2t)

pressure changes expected during the mission [22]. The concept of trapped gas also applies to respiratory medical equipment such as blood pressure cuffs, chest tube pumps, and mechanical ventilation tracheal cuffs.

Decompression Sickness

Decompression sickness (DCS) can occur due to any substantive reduction in ambient environmental pressure such as in diving, aviation, and space flight. In accordance with Henry's law, the main inert gas in solution is contingent on the ambient gas breathed by the individual and is usually nitrogen. Due to the large amount of tissue-dissolved nitrogen, a large gas load can transition into an evolved gas phase with a significant reduction in ambient pressure [23].

The signs and symptoms of DCS are classified as mild (musculoskeletal, constitutional, lymphatic, and cutaneous) or serious (cerebral, spinal cord symptoms, cardiopulmonary symptoms, cardiovascular, and inner ear symptoms) [23]. Mild symptoms manifest as musculoskeletal pain, constitutional symptoms, lymphatic, and cutaneous symptoms. Cardiopulmonary symptoms are often called "chokes" and are the result of increased bubble load within the lungs resulting in pulmonary compromise. Common symptoms include dry cough, dyspnea, and substernal chest pain. Skin bends exist either in the form of "cutis marmorata" [24] or the more serious raised, mottled truncal rash (livedo racemosa) that is suggestive of significant right-to-left shunting and often associated with worse outcomes and neurologic symptoms [25]. The timeline of hyperbaric DCS (i.e., diving) is different from hypobaric DCS (i.e., ascending altitude) due to the different tissue gas loads and ambient pressure changes. Hyperbaric DCS risk will arise after mission completion upon surfacing from higher pressure (with proportionally higher amounts of dissolved inert gas in the tissues) to ambient pressure. Hypobaric DCS risk in spaceflight will occur during the mission upon exposure to a lower ambient pressure (e.g., extravehicular activity (EVA)) compared to baseline pressure (in the space vehicle); the evolved gas load and risk are lower due to preoxygenation prior to EVA to drive down inert tissue gas load. Another important concept to keep in mind is the timing of the treatment of DCS. A diver begins experiencing symptoms toward the end of their dive, and therefore, treatment can be started immediately; however, in space, the astronaut must first return to a safe environment prior to treatment initiation, thereby resulting in treatment delays.

Evolved gas can occur commonly in the venous and rarely in the arterial systems. Usually, venous gas emboli (VGE) are filtered out through the pulmonary system and do not cause any symptoms. However, if the pulmonary system becomes oversaturated with gas bubbles (referred to as "chokes" manifesting with chest pain, shortness of breath, cough, and hypoxemia), this can lead to severe ventilation–perfusion mismatch, resulting in a large functional intrapulmonary right-to-left shunt, which causes profound hypoxemia and may progress to neurocirculatory collapse. Increased risk of paradoxical embolization (including stroke or myocardial infarction) may arise from the presence of congenital pulmonary arteriovenous malformations or intracardiac right-to-left shunting notably under conditions of increased right sided cardiac pressures (e.g., pulmonary hypertension, chronic respiratory conditions such as sleep apnea and exposure to hypoxia) and systemic vasodilatation (e.g., hypoxia). Mechanical effects can further facilitate right-to-left shunting such as coughing and the Valsalva maneuver.

A probabilistic model estimated that when exposed to 4.3 pounds per square inch absolute (PSIA) with simulated EVA (extravehicular activity = spacewalk in spacesuit at 4.3 pounds per square inch absolute (PSIA) outside of spacecraft) with ambulation after equilibration to the exploration atmosphere at 8.2 PSIA with a 34% oxygen atmosphere would result in the incidence of 3.1% DCS (1.8–5.2 95% confidence interval), 23.2% VGE (16.7–31.2%), and 8.5% Grade IV VGE (4.7–14.7%) in equal samples of men and women exposed for 6 h [26].

The extravehicular mobility unit (EMU) (Fig. 4.7) has a lower constant pressurized atmospheric pressure (4.3 PSIA) than the ISS (14.7 PSI); therefore, prior to any EVA, astronauts denitrogenate by breathing 100% oxygen, including an exercise-enhanced 100% oxygen prebreathe protocol for up to 4 h to prevent DCS [26].

Treatment options for decompression sickness during spaceflight include continued provision of 100% oxygen, return inside the spacecraft, and potential use of the EMU to increase the pressure inside the suit (4.3 PSIA) above the space station pressure (14.7 PSIA) resulting in a treatment pressure of 19 PSIA. Clinical

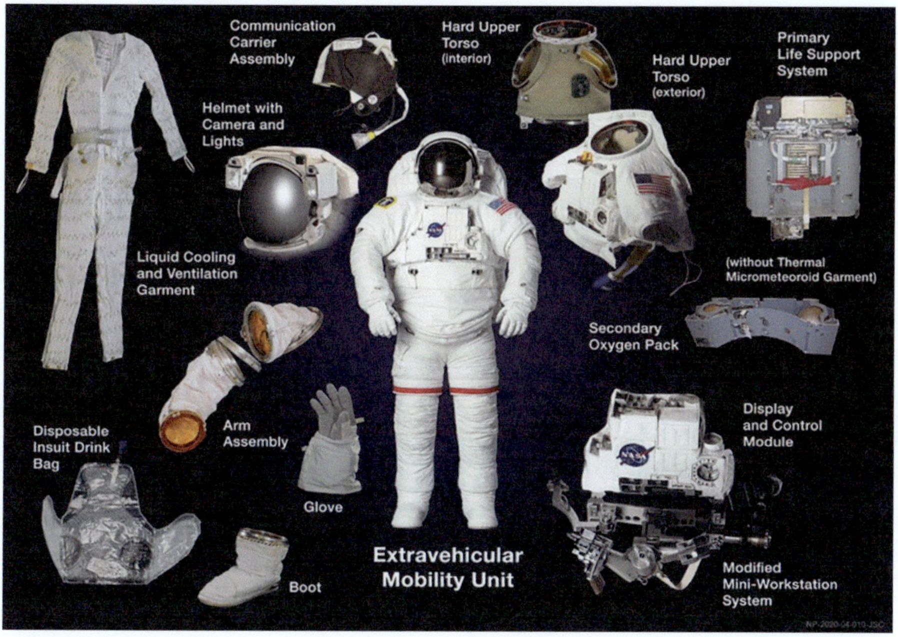

Fig. 4.7 Components and systems of the US extravehicular mobility unit (EMU). (Graphic credit: NASA)

assessment and potential extensions to stay under pressure may be advised as there is no hyperbaric chamber treatment capability beyond the in-suit bends treatment approach.

Dust Exposure

The lunar surface is layered with fine, unconsolidated material (regolith) covering solid rock, which is quite different from regolith generated on Earth through weathering mechanisms such as wind, water, ice, and biological forces. The dust on the lunar surface has been created over 4 billion years by severe temperature fluctuations, constant impact of solar wind and cosmic rays, and the mechanical effect of meteorite impacts with fragmentation of material and partial melting due to heat. These processes result in distinctly smaller particle sizes. Lunar dust is composed of particles that constitute the finest regolith with a diameter under 20 μm. Ultrafine dust is less than 1 μm, fine dust 0.1–0.5 μm, and coarse dust 2.5–10 μm. The shape of the dust is significant because of the processes creating it, including meteorite impact with shard-like glass components with jagged and very sharp edges [27]. Regolith consists of olivine, basalt, pyroxene, ilmenite, and anorthosite with the presence of iron in the form of nanophase iron (Fe^0), which raises the potential of the generation of reactive oxygen species and interference with electrical and mechanical systems of spacecraft. Experience with lunar dust exposure after extravehicular activities during Apollo 11 and subsequent Apollo missions revealed ocular and respiratory irritation after exposure events among astronauts. Astronauts also noted that the dust was very adherent to their spacesuits due to static charge. It was difficult to remove the dust despite using vacuum systems in follow-on missions. A type-4 hypersensitivity reaction of a flight surgeon repeatedly exposed to lunar dust has been reported [28]. All symptoms were self-limited and subsided within 24 h. Permissible exposure limits for lunar dust were studied by the lunar airborne dust toxicity advisory group with the recommendation in 2014 of a permissible exposure limit of 0.3 mg/m^3 for a 6-month lunar mission with 8 h of lunar dust exposure for 5 days per week be followed.

Another concern with lunar dust is the potential immunologic response to the transport of reactive particles into the terminal lung spaces. Terrestrial pneumoconiosis, such as silicosis, may serve as a model and highlight the challenge of potential prolonged timelines to appreciate alterations in pulmonary function and clinical respiratory symptoms. The combined exposures to excessive radiation [29, 30] and dust may have unforeseen deleterious effects. There are no good acute monitoring systems that would allow for serologic assessment, nor are there imaging modalities available beyond ultrasound, which for pneumoconiosis does not provide characteristic ultrasound patterns that would be of diagnostic value. Exposure prevention and mitigating risk by removing dust from habitable space or creating systems whereby dust will not enter is of paramount priority. Avoidance of polar surfaces that allow for static clinging as well as introduction of high-efficiency air filters will be of critical importance to maintain a safe and breathable atmosphere. The impact of lunar dust on other biological systems has not been well characterized, but may become more important, especially with the prolonged presence of humans on the lunar surface with potential exposure to lunar dust.

Treatment of an acute excessive exposure may necessitate supplemental oxygen, bronchodilators, and corticosteroids with consideration for an early return to earth, followed by radiological screening as well as pulmonary function testing [31].

Little is known about the pathophysiologic consequences of significant exposures to lunar dust via inhalation or the optimal technology to minimize such exposures, including the optimal suiting systems, electrostatically repulsive and particulate air filters, and magnetic filters. An occupational lung surveillance program for astronauts exposed to significant dust will be prudent and can be accomplished through the longitudinal study of astronaut health.

Infection/Altered Immunity

The environment of space flight results in documented alterations in immune function with attendant risks for infections. Atrophy of the thymus tissue has been described during space flight and is thought to be secondary to glucocorticoid stress response. Decreased activity of CD4-positive T-cells has been reported, while the activity of CD8-positive T-cells is increased during and after space flight, but with reduced function against a variety of viruses [32]. Innate immunity is accomplished through the activity of phagocytes, mainly neutrophils and monocytes, which can permeate into peripheral tissues and differentiate into macrophages. After space flight, neutrophils produce more proinflammatory cytokines when exposed to fungal antigens. During space flight, there appears to be a decreased response to macrophage colony-stimulating factor resulting in a reduction of monocyte-to-macrophage differentiation and as a result decrease in macrophage numbers documented in murine models [33]. This pattern shift of the immune response compared to the terrestrial status quo explains the increased likelihood of reactivation of herpes viruses during space flight [34].

The space flight environment is unique in that there are changes in microbial behaviors such as alterations in proliferation, virulence, capability of biofilm production, alterations in the human microbiome as well as acquisition of antibiotic resistance. Multiple factors impact alterations of microbial behavior and space such as microgravity, oscillations of temperature, cosmic radiation, and ultraviolet radiation prompting bacterial adaptive responses [30]. An analysis of bacterial and fungal species isolated inside the ISS highlighted the following as specifically concerning for human health: *Staphylococcus aureus*, *Klebsiella pneumoniae*, *Serratia marcescens*, *Bacillus*, *Mycobacterium*, and *Aspergillus* species. Microbes can adapt by altering their susceptibility to antibiotics, altering the human microbiome, creating biofilms, and increasing proliferation and virulence [35].

Measures to prevent and prophylactically manage infections during space flight include quarantine prior to spaceflight to avoid crew members carrying active infections into the space vehicle, disinfection of high touch surfaces as well as high efficiency particulate air filtration systems, sterility of water sources used for human consumption and maintenance of optimal nutrition to avoid deleterious impact on immune system function via nutritional deficiencies. Appropriate vaccinations contingent on serological data prior to prolonged space missions have proven to be beneficial in reducing varicella zoster virus reactivation during space flight and may be a viable approach to combat other emerging pathogens [35].

Microbial diagnostics during a prolonged space mission are limited based on the diagnostic modalities that are available in space flight. Antimicrobial agents have been shown to exhibit significant loss of antimicrobial activity after prolonged time in space (amoxicillin–clavulanic acid loses 50% of its potency by day 534 in space flight). Viral infections are typically self-limited, and successful treatment of a herpes simplex infection (cold sore) with valacyclovir has been reported [34, 36, 37].

The impact of the lack of gravity on the presentation and clinical course of a pulmonary infection such as a pneumonia or bronchopneumonia is not certain. A more diffuse and potentially multifocal spread may be possible in the absence of gravity compared to that seen on Earth. It is also unclear whether the effects of surface tension of mucopurulent fluids in the lungs would hamper the clearance of secretions and with that potential resolution. The relative lack of advanced medical systems and necessary medical resources that would allow management of sepsis in a long-duration space flight highlights the critical importance of preventing such a scenario.

Operational Aspects

Exploration Atmosphere

The need to complete EVA as part of lunar exploration and lunar base construction and later exploration of Mars will require the transport of life-sustaining atmospheric gases and expose astronauts to frequent decompressive stress. As discussed above under the topic of DCS, the ambient pressure that the human is exposed to will result in commensurate tissue saturation with the gas that is breathed. Given these issues, NASA investigated a combination of breathing gas concentrations and pressure that would minimize the risk of DCS while also avoiding the excess risk of fire [38]. NASA recommended and is actively investigating the creation of a novel exploration atmosphere that would allow an ambient pressure of 8.2 PSIA with 34% oxygen, resulting in an inhaled oxygen pressure of 128 mmHg using the equivalent air altitude model [39]. This ambient oxygen pressure is equivalent to the oxygen pressure that was used on 34 space shuttle missions with a pressure of 10.2 PSIA and 26.5% oxygen. This decrease in ambient living pressure will decrease the risk of DCS when transitioning into the space suit at 4.3 PSIA while breathing 100% oxygen. The equivalent altitude of 8.2 PSIA pressure and 34% oxygen using the equivalent air altitude model is 1880 m (6170 ft), which represents a mild hypobaric hypoxic exposure.

Mild hypobaric hypoxia will result in hypoxia-induced vasodilation (esp. cerebral vasculature), pulmonary arterial vasoconstriction, and a hypoxic ventilatory response (HVR) with resulting respiratory alkalosis. During space flight, concerns that may be of clinical significance include the emergence of potential acute mountain sickness secondary to hypobaric hypoxia [40] and the potential for development of spaceflight-associated neuro-ocular syndrome (SANS) with impact on vision and central nervous system function [41]. Increased cerebral vasodilation might potentially lead to an exacerbation and increased propensity for the manifestation of this syndrome. There are no data available at this juncture to either affirm or refute the impact of this proposed exploration atmosphere on this process. Added hypoxic stress due to sleep-disordered breathing does not appear to be a clinically significant concern [42]. While astronauts tend to sleep fewer hours and experience fewer hours of restorative sleep, microgravity exposure nearly eliminates most sleep-related obstructive apneas and hypopneas due to reductions in upper airway resistance. However, data regarding central sleep apnea are not available [42–44].

A separate hypothetical concern rests in the increased likelihood for right-to-left shunting caused by systemic hypoxic vasodilation and increased right heart pressures, which increase the risk of paradoxical embolization both for thrombi and arterialization of VGE. Terrestrial data have shown the importance of hypoxic stress on right-to-left shunting in clinical contexts, with some patients developing right-to-left shunting only under hypoxic conditions [45]. Clinical concern for paradoxical embolization is warranted considering the recent description of a left internal jugular vein thrombus requiring treatment with enoxaparin and apixaban during spaceflight in a female astronaut and alterations in cerebral venous outflow identified in other crew members [46–48].

EMUs

The term spacecraft is usually understood to represent the vehicle transporting crew and cargo but equally applies to the spacesuit. The key function of the spacesuit is to maintain critical life support systems that provide thermal stability and adequate breathable oxygen and remove metabolic gases and contaminants. Currently, the atmosphere of the ISS is maintained at 1 atm, composed of 21% oxygen and 78% nitrogen with trace amounts of other gases similar to sea level, but increased content of carbon dioxide (10 times higher than on Earth). The spacecraft is designed to provide a source for higher concentrations of oxygen to increase the partial pressure of oxygen. The US spacesuit worn for spacewalks outside the ISS is called the extravehicular mobility unit (EMU) (Fig. 4.7). It is designed to maintain a constant pressurized atmosphere pressure (usually around 4.3 PSI) as well as delivery of 100% oxygen and removal of carbon dioxide.

Livable Atmosphere

To maintain the well-being of its occupants, the spacecraft must supply all critical life support functions such as temperature and atmospheric pressure control, ventilation, waste management, scrubbing of metabolic waste gases, removal of volatile organic trace gases, fire detection and suppression, and water purification. The environmental control and life support system in a space vehicle is responsible for regenerative life support.

Clean water can be generated through the recycling of wastewater (i.e., crew member urine), cabin humidity condensate (i.e., crew member perspiration and respiration moisture), and water from inside the hydration system of the EVA suits. Each crew member needs about a gallon of water a day aboard the ISS for consumption, food preparation, and personal hygiene. Urine can be reclaimed and combined with other wastewater and delivered to a water processor through a series of multi-filtration beds, catalytic oxidation, and ion exchange resins for purification.

A dedicated air revitalization system maintains the atmosphere by filtering particulates and microorganisms, removal of volatile organic trace gases, and removal of carbon dioxide (CO_2). Increased CO_2 can arise in spacecraft in the absence of adequate forced air movement and may result in increased CO_2 concentrations around the head of an occupant [49]. CO_2 can be removed using thermal amine and lithium hydroxide scrubbers. Other trace contaminants and volatile gases are removed through three separate units: an activated charcoal bed, a catalytic oxidizer, and a lithium hydroxide bed.

Oxygen can be produced by applying electrolysis to water, generating oxygen and hydrogen. The oxygen is then delivered into the cabin's atmosphere for consumption, and the hydrogen is vented into space or utilized by a Sabatier reactor to convert CO_2 and hydrogen molecules into methane and water. The methane can be vented into space while the water is recycled and repurposed for crew use [50].

Assessment and Segmentation of Risk Factors

Clinicians require a global framework to approach the specific clinical risks for either healthy space flight (suborbital, orbital, lunar, and Mars) participants or those having preexisting pulmonary conditions. Important considerations centered on medical risk mitigation should factor in the unique cardiopulmonary physiologic alterations secondary to gas laws, respiratory mechanics, ventilation–perfusion relationships, lung volumes, and G-forces, among others. Awareness of specific medical threats to pulmonary function arising from such alterations within the context of the subject's flight profile and operational environment exposures informs the basic aeromedical approach for the clinician (Table 4.1). Specialists through governmental agencies and commercial spaceflight operations additionally maintain evidence-based decision-making models, regulatory medical standards, and individualized health status evaluations for prospective participants. Close collaboration between the clinician taking care of their patient and aerospace medicine providers will individualize and optimize the pulmonary health risk assessment to ensure medical safety both on the ground and beyond.

Conclusion

Physiological challenges to the pulmonary system of the human body in spaceflight are multiple, but the design of the spaceship environment (including spacesuits for EVA) has provided for the mitigation of many of these environmental stressors with well-maintained pulmonary function. The transient increases in gravitational stress during take-off and landing are well tolerated, and protective engineering measures against nominal decompressive stress prior to EVA and during spaceflight have worked well without any significant detrimental effects on pulmonary function.

There are areas of risk that have not yet been adequately characterized primarily as it pertains to long-duration missions to the Moon and Mars. Notable risks that require further study include inhalational dust exposure, prolonged radiation

Table 4.1 Pulmonary medical challenges, at-risk conditions, and environmental factors are outlined by flight profile including suborbital, low Earth orbit, lunar, and Mars missions

Flight profile		Medical challenges	At-risk conditions	Environmental factors
Suborbital		• Increased work of breathing, respiratory rate, V/Q mismatch, respiratory alkalosis, and hypoxia • Decreased vital capacity • Acceleration of atelectasis • Respiratory impairment or failure	• Structural pulmonary or small airway disease and neuromuscular or diaphragmatic disorders • Obesity and poor fitness	• Brief acceleration forces (+G_x and +G_z) • Vehicle system characteristics and flight profile
Low earth orbit	*Short duration (<48 h)*	• Hypocapnia • Altered breathing dynamics • Intrapulmonary shunting	• Restrictive, diaphragmatic, or interstitial disease • V/Q mismatch • Structural pulmonary or small airway disease, neuromuscular, or diaphragmatic disorders • Obesity and poor fitness	• Brief acceleration forces (+G_x and +G_z) • Vehicle system characteristics and flight profile • Aerosolized droplets suspended within an enclosed area
	Long duration (>48 h)	• Decompression sickness events following extravehicular activities • Increased susceptibility to acute infections or latent respiratory virus reactivation		
Lunar	*≤2 weeks*	• Respiratory impairment, fibrosis, and inflammation from lunar dust inhalation • Decompression sickness events following extravehicular activities	• Pulmonary blebs, bullae, emphysema, and asthma • Immunocompromise • Obesity and poor fitness	• Lunar dust • Micro- to partial gravity transition • Confinement within the Moon base • Lack of protective atmosphere
	>2 weeks	• High acuity pulmonary infections • Longer duration for return to definitive medical care • Radiation exposure		
Mars		• Long-term lung cancer risk from significant cosmic radiation • Inhaled Martian dust inflammatory lung changes • Increased susceptibility to acute infections or latent respiratory virus reactivation • Decompression sickness events following extravehicular activities • Rapid spread of acute respiratory illnesses	• Pulmonary blebs, bullae, emphysema, and asthma • Immunocompromise • Asymptomatic and chronic pulmonary infections (i.e., tuberculosis and Mycobacterium avium complex (MAC)) • Obesity and poor fitness	• Radiation shielding enroute • Lack of protective atmosphere • Martian dust • Micro- to partial gravity transition • Aerosolized droplets suspended within an enclosed area

Risks are not exclusive to any single flight profile but rather present the predominant factors for consideration in each category

exposure during transit to and from the destination of interest as well as while there. Last but not least, the risk of infectious disease while far away from definitive medical care and with constrained medical resources in the context of alterations of immune system function and altered virulence of microorganisms that will accompany the astronauts remains an area of concern.

A clear limitation of our knowledge rests in the fact that the vast majority of humans who experienced the physiological stressors of spaceflight have been selected to be healthy individuals without preexisting significant diseases or disabilities. This will change as we witness an ever-increasing participation of commercial civilian spaceflight participants with preexisting conditions, and it will broaden our understanding in this domain.

References

1. Maresh RW, Woodrow AD, Webb JT. Handbook of aerospace and operational physiology. 2nd ed. [cited 2025 Mar 10]. https://apps.dtic.mil/sti/citations/AD1020889.
2. Haddad M, Sharma S. Physiology, lung. In: StatPearls. Treasure Island (FL): StatPearls Publishing; 2024. [cited 2024 Dec 8]. http://www.ncbi.nlm.nih.gov/books/NBK545177/.
3. Powers KA, Dhamoon AS. Physiology, pulmonary ventilation and perfusion. In: StatPearls. Treasure Island (FL): StatPearls Publishing; 2024. [cited 2024 Dec 14]. http://www.ncbi.nlm.nih.gov/books/NBK539907/.
4. Petersson J, Glenny RW. Gas exchange and ventilation–perfusion relationships in the lung. Eur Respir J. 2014;44(4):1023–41.
5. Glenny RW. Emergence of matched airway and vascular trees from fractal rules. J Appl Physiol Bethesda Md 1985. 2011;110(4):1119–29.
6. Bhakta NR, McGowan A, Ramsey KA, et al. European Respiratory Society/American Thoracic Society technical statement: standardization of the measurement of lung volumes, 2023 update. Eur Respir J. 2023;62
7. Katz S. The effect of body position on pulmonary function: a systematic review. BMC Pulm Med. 2018;18(159):1–16.
8. Edyvean J, Estenne M, Paiva M, Engel LA. Lung and chest wall mechanics in microgravity. J Appl Physiol. 1991;71(5):1956–66.
9. Elliott AR, Prisk GK, Guy HJ, West JB. Lung volumes during sustained microgravity on Spacelab SLS-1. J Appl Physiol. 1994;77(4):2005–14.
10. Devalla L, Ghewade B, Jadhav U, Annareddy S. Resolving the complexity: a comprehensive review on carbon monoxide diffusion capacity in chronic obstructive pulmonary disease patients. Cureus. 2024;16(2):1–9, e53492.
11. Prisk GK. Microgravity and the respiratory system. Eur Respir J. 2014;43(5):1459–71.
12. Verbanck S, Larsson H, Linnarsson D, Prisk GK, West JB, Paiva M. Pulmonary tissue volume, cardiac output, and diffusing capacity in sustained microgravity. J Appl Physiol. 1997;83(3):810–6.
13. Shibata S, Wakeham DJ, Thomas JD, Abdullah SM, Platts S, Bungo MW, et al. Cardiac effects of long-duration space flight. J Am Coll Cardiol. 2023;82(8):674–84.
14. Moore TP, Thornton WE. Space shuttle inflight and postflight fluid shifts measured by leg volume changes. Aviat Space Environ Med. 1987;58(9 Pt 2):A91–6.
15. Prisk GK, Guy HJ, Elliott AR, Deutschman RA, West JB. Pulmonary diffusing capacity, capillary blood volume, and cardiac output during sustained microgravity. J Appl Physiol. 1993;75(1):15–26.

16. Buckey JC, Gaffney FA, Lane LD, Levine BD, Watenpaugh DE, Blomqvist CG. Central venous pressure in space. N Engl J Med. 1993;328(25):1853–4.
17. Videbaek R, Norsk P. Atrial distension in humans during microgravity induced by parabolic flights. J Appl Physiol. 1997;83(6):1862–6.
18. Pollock RD, Jolley CJ, Abid N, Couper JH, Estrada-Petrocelli L, Hodkinson PD, et al. Pulmonary effects of sustained periods of high-G acceleration relevant to suborbital spaceflight. Aerosp Med Hum Perform. 2021;92(7):633–41.
19. Cherniack NS, Hyde AS, Watson JF, Zechman FW. Some aspects of respiratory physiology during forward acceleration. Aerosp Med. 1961;32:113–20.
20. Pollock RD, Stevenson AT, Gates SD, Storey JA, Radcliffe JJ. Indices of acceleration atelectasis and the effect of hypergravity duration on its development. Exp Physiol. 2021;106:18–27.
21. Chen CW, Perng WC, Li MH, Yan HC, Wu CP. Hemorrhage from an enlarged emphysematous bulla during commercial air travel. Aviat Space Environ Med. 2006;77(12):1275–7.
22. Stepanek J, Blue RS, Parazynski S. Space medicine in the era of civilian spaceflight. N Engl J Med NEJM. 2019;380(11):1053–60.
23. Mitchell SJ, Bennett MH, Moon RE. Decompression sickness and arterial gas embolism. Hardin CC, editor. N Engl J Med. 2022;386(13):1254–64.
24. Conkin J, Pilmanis AA, Webb JT. Case descriptions and observations about cutis marmorata from hypobaric decompressions. Johnson Space Center: NASA; 2002. p. 1–24. Report No.: NASA/TP-2002-210779.
25. Breen I, Stepanek J, Marks L, Yale K, Mesinkovska N, Swanson D. Clinical significance of mottling rashes in diving decompression sickness. Aerosp Med Hum Perform. 2024;95(9):1–8.
26. Conkin J. Preventing decompression sickness over three decades of extravehicular activity. NASATP-2011-216147. 2011;1–34.
27. Pohlen M. Overview of lunar dust toxicity risk. Npj Microgravity. 2022;8(55):1–9.
28. Scheuring RA, Jones JA, Novak JD, Polk JD, Gillis DB, Schmid J, et al. The Apollo Medical Operations Project: recommendations to improve crew health and performance for future exploration missions and lunar surface operations. Acta Astronaut. 2008 Oct;63(7–10):980–7.
29. Simonsen LC, Slaba TC, Guida P, Rusek A. NASA's first ground-based Galactic Cosmic Ray Simulator: enabling a new era in space radiobiology research. Misteli T, editor. PLoS Biol. 2020;18(5):e3000669.
30. Tomsia M, Cieśla J, Śmieszek J, Florek S, Macionga A, Michalczyk K, et al. Long-term space missions' effects on the human organism: what we do know and what requires further research. Front Physiol. 2024;15:1284644.
31. Darquenne C, Prisk GK. Deposition of inhaled particles in the human lung is more peripheral in lunar than in normal gravity. Eur J Appl Physiol. 2008;103:687.
32. Taylor GR, Janney RP. In vivo testing confirms and blunting of the human cell mediated immune mechanism during space flight. J Leukoc Biol. 1992;51:129–1332.
33. Crucian BE, Cubbage ML, Sams CF. Altered cytokine production by specific human peripheral blood cell subsets immediately following space flight. J Interf Cytokine Res. 2000;20(6):547–56.
34. Mehta SK. Latent virus reactivation in astronauts on the international space station. Npj Microgravity. 2017;3(11):1–8.
35. Cowen D, Zhang R, Komorowski M. Infections in long-duration space missions. Lancet Microbe. 2024;5(9):100875.
36. Smith MB, Chen H, Oliver BGG. The lungs in space: a review of current knowledge and methodologies. Cells. 2024;13(1154):1–12.
37. Mehta SK. Herpes virus reactivation in astronauts during spaceflight and its application on earth. Front Microbiol. 2019;10(16)
38. Norcross J, Norsk P, Law J. Effects of the 8 psia/32% O_2 atmosphere on the human in the spaceflight environment. NASATM-2013-217377. 2013;1–44.
39. Conkin J, Wessel JH. Critique of the equivalent air altitude model. Aviat Space Environ Med. 2008;79(10):975–82.

40. West J. Physiological effects of chronic hypoxia. N Engl J Med. 2017;376:1965–71.
41. Zhang LF, Hargens AR. Spaceflight-induced intracranial hypertension and visual impairment: pathophysiology and countermeasures. Physiol Rev. 2018;98(1):59–87.
42. Elliott AR, Shea SA, Dijk DJ, Wyatt JK, Riel E, Neri DF, et al. Microgravity reduces sleep-disordered breathing in humans. Am J Respir Crit Care Med. 2001;164(3):478–85.
43. Dijk DJ, Neri DF, Wyatt JK, Ronda JM, Riel E, Ritz-De Cecco A, et al. Sleep, performance, circadian rhythms, and light-dark cycles during two space shuttle flights. Am J Physiol Regul Integr Comp Physiol. 2001;281(5):R1647–64.
44. Piltch O, Flynn-Evans EE, Young M, Stickgold R. Changes to human sleep architecture during long-duration spaceflight. J Sleep Res. 2024;34:e14345.
45. Stepanek J, Farina JM, Mahmoud AK, Chao CJ, Alsidawi S, Ayoub C, et al. Identifying the causes of unexplained dyspnea at high altitude using normobaric hypoxia with echocardiography. J Imaging. 2024;10(2):38.
46. Venous thrombosis during spaceflight. N Engl J Med. 2020;382(1):89–90.
47. Pavela J, Sargsyan A, Bedi D, Everson A, Charvat J, Mason S, et al. Surveillance for jugular venous thrombosis in astronauts. Vasc Med. 2022;27(4):365–72.
48. Wiener TC. Space obstructive syndrome: intracranial hypertension, intraocular pressure, and papilledema in space. Aviat Space Environ Med. 2012;83(1):64–6.
49. Belobrajdic B, Melone K, Diaz-Artiles A. Planetary extravehicular activity (EVA) risk mitigation strategies for long-duration space missions. Npj Microgravity. 2021;7(1):16.
50. DallBauman LA, Finn JE. Adsorption processes in spacecraft environmental control and life support systems. In: Studies in surface science and catalysis. Elsevier; 1999. p. 455–71. [cited 2024 Dec 16]. https://linkinghub.elsevier.com/retrieve/pii/S0167299199803693.

Chapter 5
Lungs at the Extremes: Lungs During Exercise

Andrew Tomlinson

Physiological Changes from Rest to Exercise

At rest at sea level, a healthy adult of average body size breathes about 10–12 times per minute on average with tidal volumes (V_T) of 400–500 mL. This results in a minute ventilation ($\dot{V}_E$) of about 4–6 L/min, sufficient to maintain a normal arterial partial pressure of CO_2 (P_aCO_2 = 35–45 mmHg). A portion of this ventilation does not participate in gas exchange due to the dead space (V_D) of the trachea and other conducting airways down to the respiratory bronchioles. The large surface area and minimal thickness (approximately 0.5–1 μm) of the alveolar-capillary interface results in efficient gas exchange and near-complete equilibration of alveolar air and end-capillary blood.

With the onset of exercise, multiple physiological changes occur. Minute ventilation increases through a combination of increasing respiratory rate and increasing tidal volume. In early exercise, this is driven more by increases in tidal volume and then later in exercise as tidal volume plateaus, by further increases in the respiratory rate. In addition to increasing overall ventilation, increasing tidal volume generally decreases V_D/V_T as anatomical dead space remains almost constant. Increases in minute ventilation serve to maintain P_aCO_2 homeostasis with increasing levels of CO_2 production from increased metabolic activity up to a ventilatory threshold and then to allow for respiratory compensation for metabolic acidosis/acidemia above that threshold. The ventilatory threshold occurs near what is sometimes called the lactate or anaerobic threshold and is typically defined by an increase in ventilation disproportionate to increasing oxygen consumption ($\dot{V}_E/\dot{V}O_2$ ratio). The increase in ventilation beyond the ventilatory threshold also serves to increase the alveolar

A. Tomlinson (✉)
University of Texas Southwestern Medical Center, Dallas, TX, USA
e-mail: andrew.tomlinson@utsouthwestern.edu

E. R. Swenson, A. M. Luks (eds.), *The Lungs at the Extremes of Environment and Age*, Respiratory Medicine, https://doi.org/10.1007/978-3-031-98371-9_5

partial pressure of oxygen (P_AO_2) and thus defend arterial oxygenation (P_aO_2) as the A-a O_2 difference increases in late exercise. The exact reasons for A-a O_2 difference increasing in late exercise are not fully understood but may relate to a combination of increased ventilation–perfusion heterogeneity, intrapulmonary shunt, possible interstitial edema, and, in highly fit endurance athletes, a diffusion limitation due to markedly decreased red blood cell capillary transit time [2].

Respiratory Mechanics

Ventilation during exercise is roughly constrained by a maximal flow-volume envelope corresponding to a maximal forced expiratory maneuver such as that obtained during spirometry. Flows at any given point within this maximal flow-volume envelope can exceed the envelope only due to a mild bronchodilation, which typically occurs during exercise as a result of sympathetic activity or due to gas compression artifact. Conversely, flow can be more constrained due to exercise-induced bronchoconstriction or emphysema and other sources of airflow obstruction. The forces required to generate the flows of a maximal flow-volume loop are generally not reached during exercise, and the entirety of the flow-volume envelope cannot be utilized. Rather, a more efficient breathing pattern is typically adopted such that by peak exercise most individuals utilize up to 50–60% of their forced vital capacity (FVC) in a range that avoids approaching both total lung capacity (where work of breathing is higher due to increased elastic recoil) and residual volume (where expiration is more flow limited). This optimization of respiratory mechanics allows for a maximal potential ventilation during exercise that roughly corresponds to about 40 times the $FEV_{1,}$ although ventilation during exercise does not typically reach this level in healthy adults other than at the extremes of physical conditioning or age. This ratio of 40 times FEV_1 is commonly used to estimate maximal voluntary ventilation (MVV) if that parameter is not directly measured (Fig. 5.1).

Pulmonary Vascular Hemodynamics

The pulmonary vascular bed in healthy individuals is a low-resistance, low-pressure circuit. During exercise as cardiac output increases, the pulmonary capillaries distend, and additional capillary beds are recruited such that pulmonary vascular pressures increase only modestly. One function of the low resistance of the pulmonary arterial system is that it allows for hypoxic and hypercapnic vasoconstriction to selectively divert blood flow away from poorly ventilated or hypoxic/hypercapnic regions of the lung. This mechanism maintains effective ventilation–perfusion matching, resulting in efficient gas exchange. Pulmonary hypertension (whether primary or secondary) blunts the effectiveness of hypoxic and hypercapnic

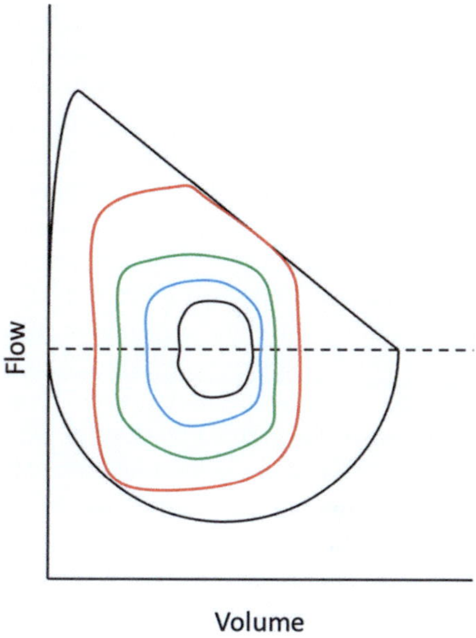

Fig. 5.1 Flow-volume loops during exercise showing progressive increase in tidal volume and flow rates from rest (black) to mild exercise (blue) to moderate exercise (green) to heavy exercise (red)

pulmonary vasoconstriction due to overall increased pulmonary vascular resistance and thus an inability to effectively redistribute pulmonary blood flow. The presence of small intrapulmonary shunts that may function to offload the pulmonary vascular system and limit increases in pulmonary vascular resistance has been debated [3], although their presence would entail the potential cost of worsening gas exchange.

Gas Exchange

The primary function of the lungs is gas exchange, allowing for the uptake of oxygen from the air and the exhalation of carbon dioxide into it. This process is accomplished efficiently by closely matching ventilation with perfusion, as referenced above. The large surface area for gas exchange and the short distance gases have to diffuse across due to the juxtaposition of the alveoli and pulmonary capillaries result in near-complete equilibration of oxygen, but less so for carbon dioxide in circumstances such as severe lung disease and heavy exercise, where a negative 2–4 mmHg alveolar to arterial PCO_2 difference may develop [4]. This has the potential to alter dead-space calculations since the Bohr–Enghoff modification of the dead-space calculation assumes $PaCO_2$ and P_ACO_2 are equal. A shortened capillary transit time due to increases in cardiac output during exercise is still generally sufficient for near-complete equilibration for oxygen to occur in healthy individuals. Factors that decrease the rate of diffusion or decrease the inspired partial pressure of oxygen (e.g., high altitude) reduce the likelihood of complete oxygen equiliibration by the end of the capillary, particularly when capillary transit time is reduced.

Efficient matching of ventilation to perfusion is primarily accomplished through differential vasoconstriction of pulmonary arterioles (including hypoxic and hypercapnic pulmonary vasoconstriction) and the historically less well-recognized effects of bronchoconstriction and reductions in local parenchymal compliance in response to decreased perfusion [5, 6]. In conjunction, these mechanisms act to limit, but not fully eliminate the effects of perturbations in regional ventilation and blood flow. In particular, bronchoconstriction and pneumoconstriction only partially decrease ventilation to a poorly perfused region of lung. Thus, areas of the lung that are poorly perfused (physiological dead space) remain at least partially ventilated resulting in wasted or excess ventilation. Ventilation of dead space does not, however, affect gas exchange as the partial pressures of gases in blood returning to the systemic circulation from the pulmonary veins are weighted by fractional blood flow through a given portion of lung. Despite the fact that it does not directly affect gas exchange, this wasted or dead-space ventilation can have physiological effects during exercise due to the increased respiratory muscle work required for ventilation.

Training/Adaptations in Elite Athletes

Impact of Cardiovascular Adaptations

Elite athletes, particularly those in endurance sports, have well-trained cardiovascular systems. Although a substantial component of cardiovascular fitness is genetically determined, training the cardiovascular system can further increase stroke volume, thus allowing increased cardiac output and increased bulk oxygen delivery to skeletal muscles. Fortunately, the pulmonary vascular system is able to accommodate this increased blood flow without substantial changes in function due to distension and recruitment of additional capillaries, which also results in a shorter transit time through the pulmonary vascular bed.

In addition to central cardiac changes from training, elite endurance athletes also undergo adaptations in the peripheral vasculature with enhanced capillarization of skeletal muscle allowing for a greater degree of oxygen extraction from blood that is delivered to exercising muscle. These adaptations result in a lower mixed venous oxygen content in the blood returning to the lungs through the right side of the heart, both due to increased oxygen extraction from blood delivered to exercising muscle and due to a greater fraction of cardiac output being delivered to exercising muscle. Again, Fortunately, the diffusing capacity of the lungs is such that, even with decreased transit time and lower mixed venous content of pulmonary arterial blood, near-complete equilibration of gases occurs, and arterial oxygen saturation is maintained to a moderate-to-high degree of training. However, in some elite athletes, hypoxemia occurs near peak exercise, a phenomenon known as exercise-induced arterial hypoxemia, which is discussed further below.

Respiratory Muscle Adaptations

While the cardiovascular system undergoes significant adaptations in response to training, the respiratory system is generally not trainable in the same way. Athletes do not develop larger lungs with training, at least not in adulthood. Swimmers generally have larger lung volumes than the average population, although it remains unclear whether this is due to selection (larger lungs make better swimmers) or a stimulus for increased lung growth from respiratory maneuvers commonly performed during swimming itself during somatic growth in adolescence. Competitive swimmers breathe in a pattern atypical for other sports with less frequent respirations at higher tidal volumes to improve stroke efficiency. Regardless, training in adulthood and in other endurance sports does not change lung size (total lung capacity or forced vital capacity) or lung function. Diffusing capacity may marginally increase, although this is likely due to an effect of increased blood volume and increased hemoglobin mass rather than changes in lung function.

Although the lungs themselves are not trainable, the muscles that control respiration are skeletal muscles capable of training to some degree. Respiratory muscle training likely results in some performance benefit, although this may be dependent on the demands required by specific sports. In most endurance sports, peak forces are not generally reached during exercise due to efficiency and constraints in the flow-volume envelope previously discussed.

Respiratory Limitations During Exercise in Elite Athletes

Elite endurance athletes are able to generate substantially higher peak cardiac outputs than untrained or sedentary subjects and thus achieve substantially higher peak oxygen consumption. They do not however significantly change their ventilatory efficiency, and thus, higher oxygen consumption ($\dot{V}O_2$) and carbon dioxide production ($\dot{V}CO_2$) necessitate a higher minute ventilation. Most untrained or sedentary subjects have significant ventilatory reserve at peak exercise, and thus, this increased ventilatory demand with training does not typically cause limitations, at least at mild-to-moderate degrees of training. However, elite athletes do reach sufficiently high levels of oxygen consumption that the minute ventilation approaches or exceeds predicted levels of maximal ventilation. This constraint to further increasing ventilation generally occurs above a ventilatory threshold and thus limits the athlete's ability to compensate for metabolic acidosis. While this could be considered to limit exercise, there are data to suggest that elite athletes actually tolerate a relatively higher P_aCO_2 and lower pH and that maximal exercise is thus still limited by the cardiovascular system rather than the respiratory system. This tolerance of a higher P_aCO_2 and lower pH may result from mild blunting of the ventilatory drive at peak exercise with repeated training. While it is not intrinsically physiologically harmful to maintain a relatively higher P_aCO_2 (above the ventilatory threshold where decreases in this would typically be expected as compensation for metabolic acidosis), this does limit the increase in alveolar PO_2, which normally limits the increase in the $(A\text{-}a)\Delta O_2$ in late exercise and may contribute to exercise-induced arterial hypoxemia. A higher P_aCO_2 within peripheral tissues may enhance off-loading of oxygen to the tissues by causing a rightward shift in the oxyhemoglobin dissociation curve.

Exercise-Induced Arterial Hypoxemia

Exercise-induced arterial hypoxemia in elite athletes is a well-recognized phenomenon for which the etiology remains unclear. In some (but not all) well-conditioned elite endurance athletes, arterial oxygen saturation falls in late exercise. This phenomenon occurs more often in female subjects and in older subjects. The primary etiology is likely increased ventilation–perfusion heterogeneity, but small intrapulmonary or extrapulmonary shunts, diffusion limitation, and relative alveolar hypoventilation may also contribute [7, 8]. The very low mixed venous oxygen content seen in elite athletes at peak exercise contributes indirectly by amplifying the effect of shunt or low $\dot{V}_a/Q$ areas (as the difference in oxygen saturation between these areas and well-ventilated areas is now larger) and by exposing diffusion limitation (as a larger change in oxygen content is needed to fully reoxygenate blood), particularly with the reduced transit time associated with increases in cardiac output [9, 10].

The degree of hypoxemia that occurs with exercise-induced arterial hypoxemia varies but can have a modest effect on limiting maximal oxygen uptake at peak exercise. Given the physiological limits on how far mixed venous oxygen content can be reduced, any reduction in arterial oxygen content at peak cardiac output would be expected to reduce maximal oxygen uptake roughly proportionately based on the principles inherent in the Fick equation:

$$\dot{V}O_2 = \dot{Q}_C \left[C_aO_2 - C_{\bar{v}}O_2\right] \tag{5.1}$$

Data in elite athletes support this hypothesis and suggest a decrease in $\dot{V}O_{2max}$ of about 1–2% for each 1% decline in oxygen saturation.

Respiratory Limitations During Exercise in Aging

Due to changes in chest wall and lung structure, lung function declines with age beginning around the third or the fourth decade of life. The chest wall stiffens as the costochondral junctions ossify, both limiting the ability of the chest wall to expand and increasing the work required to expand the chest wall. The lungs themselves become less elastic due to alveolar expansion and remodeling of the interstitial space. These changes in lung structure and function with age are further discussed in another chapter of this book on the aging lung.

These changes within the lungs and chest wall result in a progressive decline in both forced vital capacity (FVC) and forced expiratory volume in one second (FEV_1), as well as a decline in the ratio of FEV_1 to FVC due to the proportionately greater rate of decline in FEV_1 (Fig. 5.2).

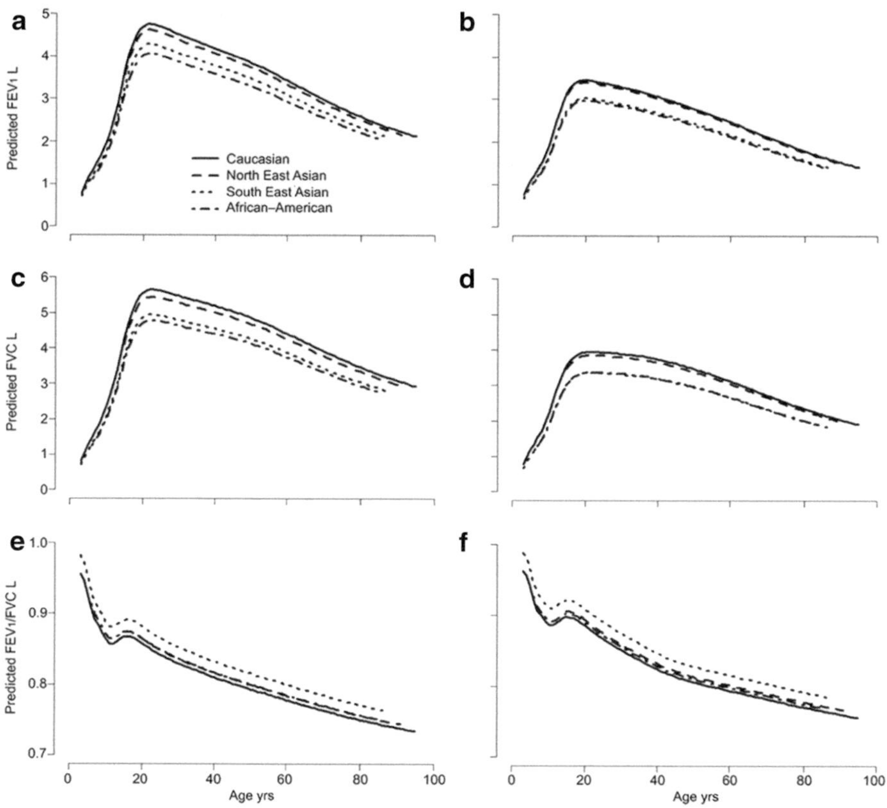

Fig. 5.2 Graphs of FEV_1 (**a**, **b**), FVC (**c**, **d**), and FEV_1/FVC ratio (**e**, **f**) for a man (**a**, **c**, **e**) and a woman (**b**, **d**, **f**) of average height across a cross-section of ages. (Reproduced from Quanjer et al. [11])

These physiological changes within the lungs have minimal impact until later life in a sedentary population given the significant ventilatory reserve typically seen with exercise in otherwise healthy individuals. With aging, a decrease in maximal heart rate and decreases in maximal stroke volume due to myocardial fibrosis also limit cardiac output. These limitations in cardiac output (and thus $\dot{V}O_{2max}$) reduce the ventilatory demand further such that a significant ventilatory reserve is generally maintained in a sedentary population until much later in life.

However, ventilation–perfusion heterogeneity does increase mildly with aging even in a healthy population. This increased ventilation–perfusion heterogeneity increases the ventilation ($\dot{V}_E$) required for a given amount of CO_2 production ($\dot{V}CO_2$) to maintain arterial CO_2 homeostasis, contributing to increased ventilatory requirements relative to maximal ventilation. Increased ventilation–perfusion heterogeneity also contributes to a widening alveolar–arterial oxygen difference with aging. Exercise-induced arterial hypoxemia occurs at a lower $\dot{V}O_2$ in a trained older population as compared to a trained younger one, likely due to both increased ventilation–perfusion heterogeneity as well as ventilatory limitations.

Changes in the FEV_1/FVC ratio and development of mild obstruction that is "normal" for advanced age result in increased expiratory flow limitation and may contribute to increased symptoms of dyspnea as ventilatory demand increases with exercise, as illustrated in Fig. 5.3.

Respiratory Limitations During Exercise in Obesity

Obesity is not thought to have a significant effect on measurements of lung function until it becomes severe (BMI >40). However, obesity of even a milder degree can influence operational lung volumes or the portion of the flow-volume envelope that is utilized during exercise. The most common initial change in pulmonary function tests with the development of obesity is a reduction in the expiratory reserve volume, thus shifting tidal volume to a portion of the flow-volume loop where more expiratory flow limitation occurs [12]. The progression of obesity subsequently results in a decrease in total lung capacity and eventually forced vital capacity, although the degree to which lung volumes are affected is variable and dependent on the distribution of adipose tissue. The effects of obesity on diffusing capacity are less clear with some data showing possible changes [13] and other data showing no change [14].

Obesity is also associated with the development of a nonallergic (non-Th2-mediated) asthma phenotype, particularly affecting the small airways. The effects of airflow obstruction associated with this are amplified by the concomitant shift in operating lung volumes toward residual volume induced by obesity.

In addition to the increased work of locomotion with obesity, obesity also has significant effects on the work of breathing during exercise due to the increased inspiratory work required to move a heavier chest wall and to displace abdominal fat [15–17]. Likely because of this increased work, ventilatory equivalents ($\dot{V}_E/\dot{V}O_2$)

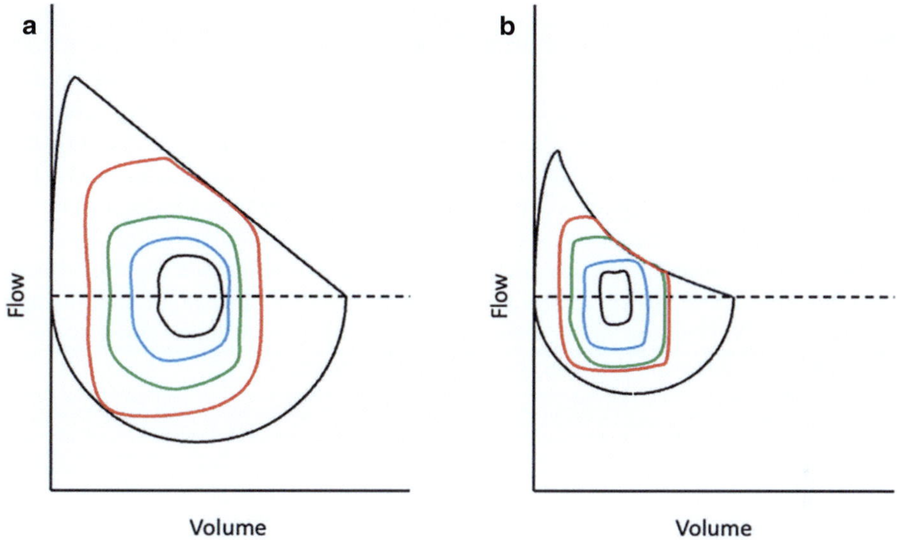

Fig. 5.3 Flow-volume loops of healthy normal 30-year-old (Panel **a**) versus healthy normal 80-year-old (Panel **b**) during exercise (rest—black; low intensity—blue; moderate intensity—green; high intensity—red). Note the smaller forced vital capacity with age, development of scooping of the expiratory portion of the flow-volume loop, and more prominent expiratory flow limitation

tend to be lower with obesity as ventilation is relatively constrained [18]. Obese patients may also have a higher arterial CO_2 setpoint (including due to obesity hypoventilation syndrome), thus reducing ventilatory requirements. However, reduced ventilation (either due to constraint or due to a higher arterial CO_2 set point) will result in a lower alveolar partial pressure of oxygen and thus a higher risk of hypoxemia during exercise.

Respiratory Limitations During Exercise at High Altitudes

While exercise at sea level is not commonly limited by the respiratory system in healthy individuals, exercise at high altitudes poses significant demands on the respiratory system. The primary difference at high altitudes is a reduced atmospheric partial pressure of oxygen due to the lower barometric pressure. The reduced inspired partial pressure of oxygen results in hypoxemia, which the respiratory system partially compensates for by increasing minute ventilation. This is effective at maintaining arterial oxygen saturation at low and modest levels of altitude but is incapable of effectively maintaining saturation at extreme high altitudes [19]. While increasing minute ventilation raises arterial oxygen saturation beyond what would be found in the absence of hyperventilation, this increased ventilation [20] comes at the cost of decreased ventilatory reserve and increased respiratory muscle oxygen consumption for a given level of work. At higher workloads, increased respiratory muscle oxygen consumption results in the diversion of a significant enough portion of blood flow to affect oxygen delivery to the muscles being used for mechanical work [21]. Furthermore, other changes including hypoxic pulmonary vasoconstriction result in a worsening of ventilation–perfusion mismatch at high altitudes [22]. When mixed venous oxygen content decreases during exercise at high altitudes (similar to sea level), the combination of a lower alveolar partial pressure of oxygen and thus a lower driving pressure for diffusion, as well as decreased capillary transit time due to increased cardiac output, results in an effective diffusion limitation and hypoxemia [23]. The use of supplemental oxygen at high altitudes easily corrects this as a larger diffusion gradient for oxygen is restored.

Summary

The respiratory system does not typically limit exercise in healthy adults. However, in various states, including in the extremes of physical conditioning, age, body habitus, and elevation, the respiratory system may at least contribute to exercise limitation. Each of these conditions results in either a decrease in lung function or an increase in the physiological demands on the lung, thus reducing the buffer of excess ventilatory reserve that typically exists. One particular example is the phenomenon of exercise-induced arterial hypoxemia, which nicely illustrates the physiologic limits of lung function.

References

1. Dempsey JA, La Gerche A, Hull JH. Is the healthy respiratory system built just right, overbuilt, or underbuilt to meet the demands imposed by exercise? J Appl Physiol (1985). 2020;129(6):1235–56. https://doi.org/10.1152/japplphysiol.00444.2020. Epub 2020 Aug 13. PMID: 32790594; PMCID: PMC7864246.
2. Lovering AT, Haverkamp HC, Eldridge MW. Responses and limitations of the respiratory system to exercise. Clin Chest Med. 2005;26(3):439–57, vi. https://doi.org/10.1016/j.ccm.2005.05.005. PMID: 16140137.
3. Stickland MK, Tedjasaputra V, Seaman C, Fuhr DP, Collins SÉ, Wagner H, van Diepen S, Byers BW, Wagner PD, Hopkins SR. Intra-pulmonary arteriovenous anastomoses and pulmonary gas exchange: evaluation by microspheres, contrast echocardiography and inert gas elimination. J Physiol. 2019;597(22):5365–84. https://doi.org/10.1113/JP277695. Epub 2019 Sep 26. PMID: 31429918; PMCID: PMC6858494.
4. Swenson ER. The pathway for carbon dioxide: from tissues to lungs. In: Joyner M, Dempsey J, editors. On oxygen: from air to tissues. Amsterdam: Elsevier Publishers. p. 221–8.
5. Swenson ER. The unappreciated role of carbon dioxide in ventilation/perfusion matching. Anesthesiology. 2019;131(2):226–8. https://doi.org/10.1097/ALN.0000000000002791. PMID: 31107277.

6. Langer T, Castagna V, Brusatori S, Santini A, Mauri T, Zanella A, Pesenti A. Short-term physiologic consequences of regional pulmonary vascular occlusion in pigs. Anesthesiology. 2019;131(2):336–43. https://doi.org/10.1097/ALN.0000000000002735. PMID: 31094756.
7. Dempsey JA, Wagner PD. Exercise-induced arterial hypoxemia. J Appl Physiol (1985). 1999;87(6):1997–2006. https://doi.org/10.1152/jappl.1999.87.6.1997. PMID: 10601141.
8. Hopkins SR. The lung at maximal exercise: insights from comparative physiology. Clin Chest Med. 2005;26(3):459–68, vi. https://doi.org/10.1016/j.ccm.2005.05.003. PMID: 16140138.
9. Hopkins SR, Dempsey JA, Stickland MK. Capillary red cell transit time is an important contributor to exercise-induced pulmonary diffusion limitation. Med Sci Sports Exerc. 2024;56(8):1538–41. https://doi.org/10.1249/MSS.0000000000003428. Epub 2024 Mar 29. PMID: 38555487; PMCID: PMC11250699.
10. Piiper J, Scheid P. Model for capillary-alveolar equilibration with special reference to O_2 uptake in hypoxia. Respir Physiol. 1981;46(3):193–208. https://doi.org/10.1016/0034-5687(81)90121-3. PMID: 6798659.
11. Quanjer PH, Stanojevic S, Cole TJ, Baur X, Hall GL, Culver BH, Enright PL, Hankinson JL, Ip MS, Zheng J, Stocks J, ERS Global Lung Function Initiative. Multi-ethnic reference values for spirometry for the 3-95-yr age range: the global lung function 2012 equations. Eur Respir J. 2012;40(6):1324–43. https://doi.org/10.1183/09031936.00080312. Epub 2012 Jun 27. PMID: 22743675; PMCID: PMC3786581.
12. Babb TG. Exercise ventilatory limitation: the role of expiratory flow limitation. Exerc Sport Sci Rev. 2013;41(1):11–8. https://doi.org/10.1097/JES.0b013e318267c0d2. PMID: 23038244; PMCID: PMC3529766.
13. Saydain G, Beck KC, Decker PA, Cowl CT, Scanlon PD. Clinical significance of elevated diffusing capacity. Chest. 2004;125(2):446–52. https://doi.org/10.1378/chest.125.2.446. PMID: 14769723.
14. Holley AB, Carbone T, Holtzclaw AW, Huprikar NA, Wagner R, Morris MJ. Obesity-related changes in diffusing capacity and transfer coefficient of the lung for carbon monoxide and resulting patterns of abnormality across reference equations. Ann Am Thorac Soc. 2023;20(7):969–75. https://doi.org/10.1513/AnnalsATS.202207-640OC. PMID: 36763964.
15. Bernhardt V, Babb TG. Exertional dyspnoea in obesity. Eur Respir Rev. 2016;25(142):487–95. https://doi.org/10.1183/16000617.0081-2016. PMID: 27903669; PMCID: PMC9487557.
16. Lorenzo S, Babb TG. Ventilatory responses at peak exercise in endurance-trained obese adults. Chest. 2013;144(4):1330–9. https://doi.org/10.1378/chest.12-3022. PMID: 23722607; PMCID: PMC3787919.
17. Bernhardt V, Wood HE, Moran RB, Babb TG. Dyspnea on exertion in obese men. Respir Physiol Neurobiol. 2013;185(2):241–8. https://doi.org/10.1016/j.resp.2012.10.007. Epub 2012 Oct 17. PMID: 23085240; PMCID: PMC3529969.
18. Balmain BN, Halverson QM, Tomlinson AR, Edwards T, Ganio MS, Babb TG. Obesity blunts the ventilatory response to exercise in men and women. Ann Am Thorac Soc. 2021;18(7):1167–74. https://doi.org/10.1513/AnnalsATS.202006-746OC. PMID: 33465334; PMCID: PMC8328370.
19. West JB, Boyer SJ, Graber DJ, Hackett PH, Maret KH, Milledge JS, Peters RM Jr, Pizzo CJ, Samaja M, Sarnquist FH, et al. Maximal exercise at extreme altitudes on Mount Everest. J Appl Physiol Respir Environ Exerc Physiol. 1983;55(3):688–98. https://doi.org/10.1152/jappl.1983.55.3.688. PMID: 6415008.
20. Pugh LG, Gill MB, Lahiri S, Milledge JS, Ward MP, West JB. Muscular exercise at great altitudes. J Appl Physiol. 1964;19:431–40. https://doi.org/10.1152/jappl.1964.19.3.431. PMID: 14173539.
21. Harms CA, Babcock MA, McClaran SR, Pegelow DF, Nickele GA, Nelson WB, Dempsey JA. Respiratory muscle work compromises leg blood flow during maximal exercise. J Appl Physiol (1985). 1997;82(5):1573–83. https://doi.org/10.1152/jappl.1997.82.5.1573. PMID: 9134907.

22. Wagner PD, Sutton JR, Reeves JT, Cymerman A, Groves BM, Malconian MK. Operation Everest II: pulmonary gas exchange during a simulated ascent of Mt. Everest. J Appl Physiol (1985). 1987;63(6):2348–59. https://doi.org/10.1152/jappl.1987.63.6.2348. PMID: 3436869.
23. Hopkins SR. Exercise induced arterial hypoxemia: the role of ventilation-perfusion inequality and pulmonary diffusion limitation. Adv Exp Med Biol. 2006;588:17–30. https://doi.org/10.1007/978-0-387-34817-9_3. PMID: 17089876.

Chapter 6
Comparative Lung Physiology at Environmental Extremes

Catherine M. Ivy

The respiratory system of vertebrates exhibits similarities despite their diverse forms. With the evolution of multicellularity and aerobic respiration came the need for specialized structures for efficient gas exchange [1, 2]. Specific metabolic requirements resulted in further natural selection on gas exchangers [3], resulting in the diversity we see today. This diversity includes the skin for cutaneous diffusion (in some amphibians), gills (some amphibians and fish), and lungs (amphibians, reptiles, birds, and mammals), all with the primary function of gas exchange. Although morphologically different, these structures have a set of common characteristics: a large capillary network, thin and moist gas exchange surfaces, constant renewal of oxygen-rich fluid (air or water) to provide oxygen and remove carbon dioxide, and free movement of blood within the capillary network [1, 4]. This chapter will focus on respiratory system anatomy and physiology among different vertebrate groups and highlight the responses of gas exchange systems in extreme environments. The reader is encouraged to seek out further reading on the complexities of breathing (neural control and peripheral and central chemosensing) in a variety of vertebrate taxa, to complement this chapter [5–9].

The original version of the chapter has been revised. A correction to this chapter can be found at https://doi.org/10.1007/978-3-031-98371-9_9

C. M. Ivy (✉)
Department of Biology, University of Saskatchewan, Saskatoon, SK, Canada
e-mail: catherine.ivy@usask.ca

E. R. Swenson, A. M. Luks (eds.), *The Lungs at the Extremes of Environment and Age*, Respiratory Medicine, https://doi.org/10.1007/978-3-031-98371-9_6

Fishes

The Fundamentals of Gills

Gill structures in aquatic vertebrates have evolved to optimize O_2 extraction and CO_2 excretion in a medium that contains significantly less O_2 than air, but a higher solubility for CO_2. Gills are the main respiratory organ in fish and some amphibians, with gas exchange occurring via passive diffusion across the respiratory epithelium of the lamellae, plate-like structures that project out of the gill filaments (Fig. 6.1a). To breathe, water enters through the mouth and out through the gills, a direction that is opposite to the flow of blood in the gill [10, 11], allowing for a constant renewal of O_2 to contact the respiratory surfaces. This counter-current design allows for 80–90% of dissolved oxygen in water to be extracted [1, 11]. Similar to the mammalian lung, not all lamellae are perfused under resting conditions, with perfusion modulated by hormones and neurotransmitters to support gas exchange during hypoxia, exercise, or other stressors [6, 12]. It is important to note that gills are a multifunctional organ and contribute to osmoregulation, metabolic acid–base regulation, and excretion of nitrogenous wastes [10, 13], in addition to gas exchange.

In water-breathing fishes, total gill ventilation can be modulated in response to changes in oxygen supply and/or demand, altering the amount of water moved across the gills per unit time [14]. Changes in gill ventilation amplitude alone, or with ventilation frequency, are commonly observed [15], as they are the least energetically costly changes that enhance ventilation in the dense, viscous medium of water [15]. Some fishes will also employ ram ventilation, where they swim with their mouth agape, passively increasing the flow of water over the gills. In obligate ram ventilators, like pelagic sharks and tunas, increases in swim speed and mouth gape aid in increasing ventilation [16]. Additionally, some fish can employ aquatic surface respiration, where they skim O_2-rich water near the air–water interface, enhancing the 'quality' of water over the gills [17].

Structural Changes in Gills

Exercise

There is a wide diversity of fishes, so it is no surprise that there is large variation in gill structure and ventilation patterns that can be linked to metabolism and environment. There is no set number of lamellae on a filament, and the total number of lamellae can be influenced by filament length, lamellar density, and lamellar length (Fig. 6.1b). Thickness of the epithelium of the lamellae can also vary, with active species having thinner epithelia than sedentary species, allowing for a shorter distance for O_2 to travel to the blood [14]. In the tuna, a fast-growing species with a high metabolic rate, the respiratory (lamellar) surface area relative to body weight

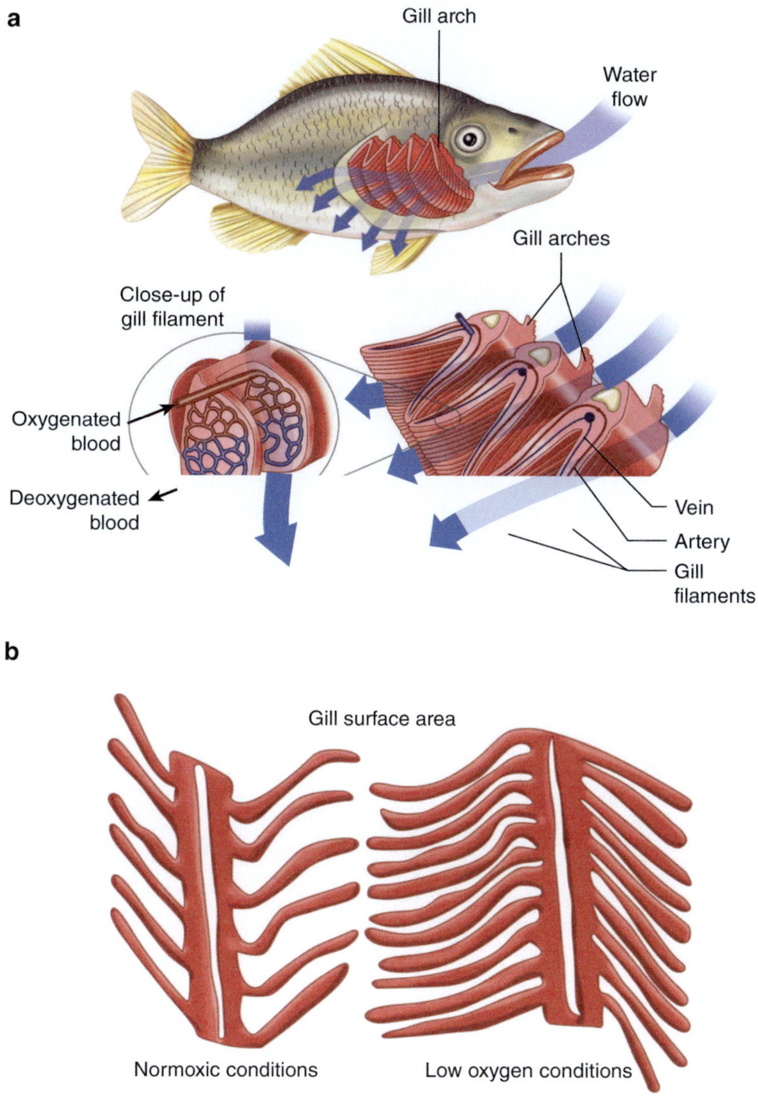

Fig. 6.1 The fish gill is a counter-current system. Fish drink water which is excreted through the gills; the volume and frequency of water movement over the gills can be adjusted to support oxygen demand (**a**). Gill filaments and lamellae can also adjust to environmental extremes over various timeframes, with changes in lamellar length, density, and thickness (**b**)

can be up to ten times greater than other ray-finned fishes (i.e. teleosts) and is similar to that found in mammals [18, 19]. Many modifications to the tuna gill have occurred to support its high metabolic rate, including thinner lamellae than other teleosts (approximately one-tenth), shorter lamellae to reduce resistance to water flow, and a high lamellar density [19, 20]. Due to their fast-swimming speeds, the lamellae are fused at the distal end to resist mechanical deformation with high water flow across the gills [20, 21]. These modifications to gill structure are in contrast to those observed in deep-sea fishes, which have low metabolic rates and a sluggish lifestyle [22]. The ventilation rate of deep-sea fishes is very slow, with Chaunacids ventilating once every 1–4 min, but having a high-volume gill ventilatory cycle compared to other teleosts [23].

Temperature and O_2 Availability

Oxygen solubility in water is influenced by water temperature, with warmer water having lower solubility compared to colder water, which can influence the ability of a fish to balance gas exchange and osmoregulation [24, 25]. Lab experiments focused on constant hypoxic (low-dissolved O_2) waters have shown that water-breathing fishes exhibit a mixture of responses in gill structure remodelling. Some species, such as freshwater carp (*Cyprinus carpio*), increase gill surface area through longer gill filaments to enhance O_2 uptake [26], but at the cost of increased ion loss. Arctic char (*Salvelinus alpinus*), rainbow trout (*Oncorhynchus mykiss*), and killifish (*Fundulus heteroclitus*), in contrast, decrease gill surface area through shorter gill filaments in an effort to reduce ion disruption [27–29]. Why some fishes exhibit one strategy over another is not well understood, but may be influenced by the ability of the gill epithelium to transition towards a less ion-permeable morphology [30].

Experiments focusing on fishes found in Antarctic and Amazonian waters have highlighted how fish have altered breathing and gill structures in response to temperature and dissolved O_2 availability. In the Antarctic, water temperatures range between −2 and 4 °C with a high-dissolved O_2 content. Icefish, a subgroup of notothenioid fishes, are benthic fish that have a low metabolic rate due to cold temperatures. The high-dissolved O_2 content of the water and low metabolism of these fishes allow them to have minimal modifications in their gill structures, such that they are similar to non-Antarctic dwelling fishes, but have larger blood vessels perfusing the gills [31]. Increased perfusion of the gills is important, as these fish have lost the O_2-transporting protein haemoglobin [32], so O_2 is dissolved in the blood plasma for transport to the tissues as the only transport form of O_2 [33].

In contrast, the Amazon River is characterized by warm water temperatures and low-dissolved O_2 content. Water-breathing fish in the Amazon River, such as the Amazonian oscar (*Astronotus ocellatus*), have suppressed metabolism (reduced O_2 demands) to match their O_2-poor environment [34]. This metabolic suppression has driven their survival, as they do not exhibit changes in gill filament or lamellae structures compared to other teleost fish [35], despite being able to remodel their gill epithelium over a short hypoxic exposure [28], and they have a similar hypoxic ventilatory response to other Amazonian and neotropical fishes [34, 36, 37]. Other fish species in the Amazon have evolved the ability to breathe air, either obligatorily (air-breathe regardless of the amount of dissolved O_2) or facultatively (when there is insufficient dissolved O_2). Obligate air-breathers either use a rudimentary paired lungs, such as the South American lungfish (*Lepidosiren paradoxa*), or a modified swim bladder that resembles a lung, as in *Arapaima* [38], both being highly vascularized for O_2 uptake. Alternatively, the gills of these species are reduced and have low-diffusion capacity, due to short lamellae with thick epitheliums, but still play a critical role in ion regulation and are ventilated in water [38–40]. The skin also plays an important role in O_2 and CO_2 diffusion, with a large proportion of CO_2 eliminated across the skin when in water [38–41]. In facultative air-breathing fish, the stomach, intestine, mouth, and pharynx are highly vascularized to take up O_2 from the air, while the gills are the primary site for O_2 uptake when in normoxic water [42]. O_2 supply and demand therefore plays an important role in the morphology and use of gills in fishes.

Amphibians and Reptiles

The transition from an aquatic environment to a terrestrial one brought organisms into an environment rich in O_2, but with the challenges of water balance and disposing of CO_2 [1], among other physiological functions [43, 44]. Respiratory structures were internalized for protection, especially from dehydration as these surfaces are highly vascularized and saturated with water, resulting in high water-loss rates [45]. To avoid respiratory acidosis, some species increased reliance on the skin for CO_2 removal, resulting in a thinner epithelium and reductions in scales [1]. Enhanced bicarbonate buffering in the blood also helped compensate for increased CO_2 levels [1]. This transition to land resulted in variation in lung morphology that matches the environment and metabolic demands of the organism.

Amphibians

Amphibians exhibit a wide range of respiratory surface morphologies due to the diversity of environments they inhabit, low metabolic rate, and patterns of interrupted development. They often inhabit moist environments, as they rely heavily on staying hydrated due to their high susceptibility to desiccation [45]. As tadpoles, they depend on gills for gas exchange, but upon metamorphosis they use lungs, skin, and mouth (buccal gas exchange) for respiration [1] (Fig. 6.2). Cutaneous respiration has been shown to fully support metabolism when amphibians are at rest [45–48]. When amphibians are in an aquatic or moist environment, the cost of cutaneous gas exchange is low compared to water loss (unlike in dry environments)

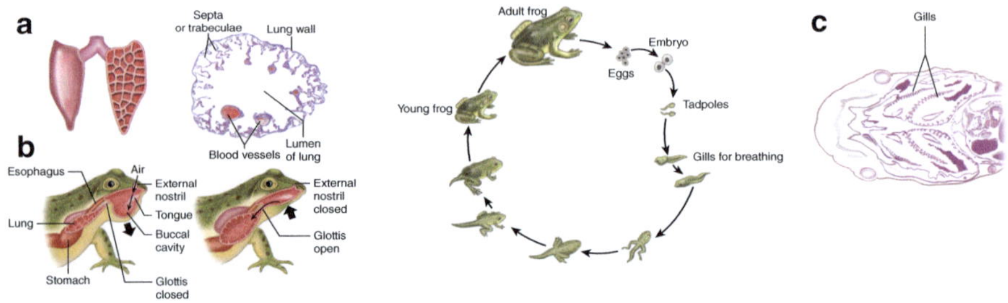

Fig. 6.2 Amphibians have varying life stages that use different respiratory structures. As adults, frogs have a simple lung (**a**) that is ventilated via buccal pumping (**b**), with the ability to respire cutaneously. In contrast, tadpoles rely on skin and gills as they develop lungs (**c**)

[45], thereby making it overall more cost-effective compared to lung ventilation, although less efficient [45]. As with fish gills and the mammalian lung, perfusion of the vasculature in the skin can be regulated, controlling gas exchange and water loss [45, 47]. The majority of adult amphibians have simple, rudimentary paired lungs with interconnected folds and varying subdivisions, depending on the species and the extent of gas exchange performed by the lungs in conjunction with cutaneous and buccal gas exchange [49]. Since amphibians lack ribs or a diaphragm, their pulmonary ventilation is driven by swallowing air through the rising of the oral cavity floor [50] (Fig. 6.2a).

Structural Changes in Respiratory Surfaces

Environment and Exercise

Three major taxa (orders) comprise Amphibia: Gymnophiona (limbless caecilians), Caudata or Urodela (newts and salamanders), and Anura (frogs and toads), with adults having varying lung complexity. Caecilians are limbless amphibians that are found in soil and streambeds with a subterranean and low metabolic lifestyle. Although caecilians can rely on cutaneous respiration, they possess long, tubular lungs that are subdivided internally to form air cells, and sometimes the left lung can be reduced or missing [51]. Not much is known about these species due to their cryptic lifestyle. Similar to caecilian amphibians, urodele amphibians (newts and salamanders) are found in moist environments and have simple paired lungs that are poorly vascularized due to their high reliance on skin and buccal cavity gas exchange [52]. The lungs have been completely lost in some salamanders found in cold, well-aerated water, with gas exchange only occurring across the skin and buccal cavity [52]. These lungless salamanders have significantly lower maximal O_2 consumption during exercise and lower maximal speed compared to lunged salamanders [53], highlighting how lifestyle and environment can modulate respiratory physiology.

Anurans (frogs and toads) have the most complex lungs of all amphibians, which may be due to the diversity in adult habitat (ranging from fully aquatic to fully terrestrial). Anuran lungs are paired and divided into small air cells (Fig. 6.2b). Lung and skin morphology in anurans is highly dictated by environment and metabolic rate. Toads, which have a higher metabolic rate and a more terrestrial lifestyle, have larger lung volumes with greater capillary density compared to the skin, and higher pulmonary surface area and compliance compared to fully aquatic frogs [54–57]. Aquatic hypoxia can also alter respiratory gas exchange surfaces in frogs, with tadpoles reared in hypoxic conditions having thicker skin, increased gill thickness, and increased lung growth to support aerial respiration and reduce aquatic gas exchange [58]. Adjustments in skin, gills, and lung development do not occur when tadpoles are reared in hyperoxia, and there are no differences in the skin or lungs of adult frogs when they are exposed to hypoxia or hyperoxia as tadpoles [58]. These findings in adult frogs are in contrast to anurans found at high altitude, which have significantly smaller lungs compared to frogs found at sea level and excessive skin area, which is presumed to enhance cutaneous gas exchange [56, 59].

Reptiles

In contrast to amphibians, reptiles rely solely on their lungs for respiration due to their thicker epidermis, which is adapted to prevent dehydration [60]. There is a large amount of heterogeneity in reptilian lung structures, which can be grouped into three types: (1) the unicameral lung, which is a saccular, smooth-walled, and transparent lung found in teju lizards; (2) the paucicameral lung, which contains subdivisions but is simpler than the multicameral lung and is found in chameleons and iguanids; and (3) the multicameral lung, which has many subdivisions and is found in turtles, monitor lizards, crocodiles, and snakes [61] (Fig. 6.3). Increases in respiratory surface area are associated with higher metabolic rates in reptiles [56], as there is a greater pulmonary diffusive capacity for O_2 [62]. Regardless of lung type, reptiles lack a diaphragm and use their ribs and intercostal muscles to effectively ventilate their lungs [63, 64].

Hypoxia

Few studies have examined how environmental hypoxia influences lung structure and breathing in reptiles. Environmental hypoxia has been shown to influence lung vasculature in reptiles, with acute hypoxia causing vasoconstriction but only in reptiles with complex lungs, which are more prone to ventilation–perfusion mismatch [62]. Some temperate reptile species, such as snapping turtles and garter snakes, are capable of withstanding severe hypoxia to anoxia, but this is due to reductions in metabolism and not modification to lung structure or breathing (reviewed in [65]).

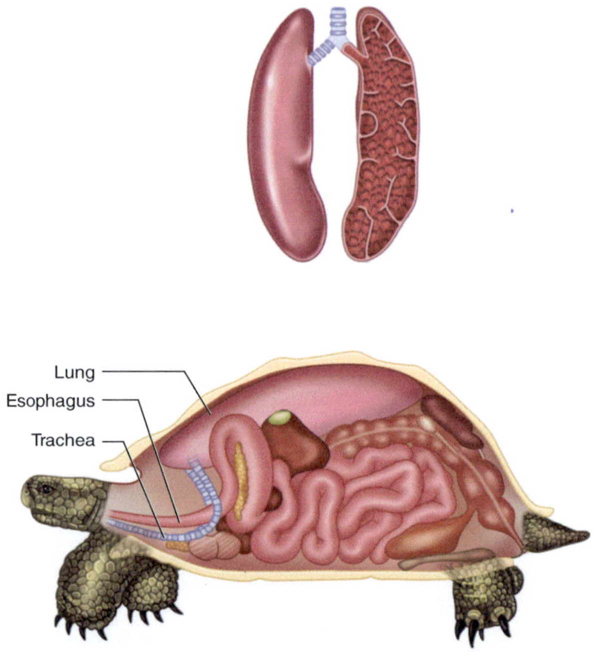

Fig. 6.3 Reptile lungs, such as those of tortoises, are more saccular with greater respiratory surface area compared to amphibians. Due to the lack of a diaphragm, the lungs are ventilated via rib and intercostal muscle movements

Diving

Sea turtles exhibit evolutionary adaptations in lung structure and breathing that allow them to cope with increased pressures during dives and brief surfacing periods for gas exchange. In contrast to other reptiles that live in shallow-water environments, the lungs of sea turtles have strongly reinforced intrapulmonary bronchi with large diameters and fibrous connective tissue to prevent collapse during dives [64, 66, 67]. These adaptations enable high ventilatory flows during brief resurfacing periods, with low airway resistance and strong muscular contributions for rapid, effective ventilation similar to diving marine mammals [66, 68, 69]. Similarly, sea turtles have larger lung volumes and deeper tidal volumes compared to other terrestrial turtles [70–72].

Mammals

The evolution of homeothermy in mammals and birds resulted in high rates of O_2 uptake, supported by a large gas exchange surface area [1]. Although many physiological systems are similar between mammals and birds, the respiratory system is quite different and highlights the increased demand for gas exchange that is further associated with different modes of locomotion [73]. The mammalian lung is thought to have evolved from the multicameral lung found in reptiles [49]. The addition of a diaphragm aids inspiration, while abdominal wall muscles aid expiration [74], although the lungs do not empty completely during respiration [75]. As most of this book is dedicated to the human (mammalian) lung, only some choice adaptations of mammalian lungs at extremes have been highlighted.

High-Altitude Hypoxia

When mammals encounter hypoxia (either environmental or due to medical conditions), various physiological responses occur to maintain oxygen uptake. As described earlier for mammals residing at sea-level altitudes (Chapter 3), changes in breathing pattern can be important for maintaining O_2 supply, while the lungs themselves can exhibit regional pulmonary vasoconstriction to aid in ventilation–perfusion matching. These responses are not as beneficial when in high-altitude hypoxia. For many mammals that live at high altitude where hypoxia is unremitting, adaptations at the level of O_2 uptake and the lung have occurred. Many high-altitude rodents, such as deer mice (*Peromyscus maniculatus*) found in the Rocky Mountains in the United States, are known to take slower, deeper breaths compared to lowland populations [76]. Additionally, some high-altitude-adapted mammals also experience minimal pulmonary vasoconstriction [77–81], maintaining large amounts of surface area available for gas exchange. This is thought to be due to dysfunctional and/or downregulation of potassium voltage-gated (Kv) channels in the pulmonary artery smooth muscles [82] and minimal muscularization of the pulmonary arteries, which are observed in plateau pika (*Ochotona curzoniae*), yaks (*Bos grunniens*), and llamas (*Lama glama*) [78, 79, 81, 82].

Diving

Deep-diving mammals, such as pinnipeds (seals) and cetaceans (whales, dolphins, and porpoises), exhibit adaptations that allow for diving to depths over 30 m, where alveolar collapse can occur [83–85]. As mentioned earlier (Chapter 2), descent to and ascent from deep-dive depths can influence the dissolved gases in the body and can be harmful to divers. Deep-diving pinnipeds and cetaceans have overcome these challenges through various adaptations. Due to increasing pressure with dive depth, the lung cannot be relied on as an O_2 store in deep-diving species. Instead, these species have smaller lungs compared to shallow-diving species [83, 85–89], with altered compliance and elasticity to support alveolar collapse [83, 85, 90, 91]. The conducting airways have cartilaginous reinforcement to prevent compression of the airway, with some species having reinforcement all the way down to the entrance of the alveoli or alveolar sacs [92]. Deep-diving species therefore use splenic blood reserves, which are highly oxygenated and viscous blood reserves, that are released into circulation when O_2 levels fall during dives [93]. These species ultimately have larger blood volume, and higher haematocrit, and haemoglobin and myoglobin concentrations compared to shallow-diving species [94].

Flight

Flight is the most energetically expensive form of exercise, up to two times or more expensive than running [95]. Bats provide a unique opportunity to explore how the mammalian lung has been adapted to support flight, which has not evolved in any other mammalian taxa, highlighting the constraints that the tidal design employs on the upper limits of mammalian exercise capacity. Bat lungs have been shown to be larger than expected for their body size [96, 97] with relatively large respiratory surface area (through wider alveoli), lower surface density of alveoli, a thinner blood–gas barrier, and a greater pulmonary capillary blood volume compared to non-flying mammals [98]. These modifications in lung structure allow for a high pulmonary diffusing capacity, supporting an O_2 uptake capacity during flight that is equivalent to that of birds [98]. Furthermore, these changes are complemented by adaptations in other steps of the O_2 cascade (e.g. cardiac output, haematology, and O_2 transport to the flight muscles [98–101]). Despite these adaptations, it is suggested that the energetically demanding aspects of flight and the inefficient tidally-ventilated mammalian lung have restricted the upper limit of the size of bats, as birds can be up to a magnitude larger in size compared to the largest bat [98].

Birds

The avian lung is the most complex and efficient gas exchanger, critical for supporting thermoregulation and high metabolic rates. Birds maintain a higher body temperature compared to most mammals (40–42 °C, although mammalian temperature can range between 36 and 40 °C) and have an overall higher metabolic rate compared to mammals of the same body mass [102–104]. Their lungs have also been adapted to support flight, which is the most costly form of locomotion [95, 102, 105], with migratory flight occurring for multiple hours to days before birds stop and rest.

The avian respiratory system is an air sac system, involving a paired lung/parabronchi (gas exchange site) uncoupled from compliant, non-respiratory air sacs (ventilatory part) [102] (Fig. 6.4). The lung is highly efficient due to the cross-current design, with continuous and unidirectional parabronchial ventilation [61] and large respiratory surface areas with a thin blood–gas barrier [98]. Instead of alveoli, birds have air capillaries that are 'labyrinthic' compared to the monopodial branching observed in mammals [102, 106]. These air capillaries are surrounded by blood capillaries, which have a very thin blood–gas barrier and are more rigid compared to capillaries found in mammalian lungs [102, 107, 108]. These rigid capillaries result in minimal/absent pulmonary vasoconstriction compared to the mammalian lung [109–113]. Blood flows in the opposite direction of airflow through the lungs [102, 108], resulting in high gas exchange. As birds do not have a diaphragm, the lungs are closely attached to the ribs and vertebrae [11, 102], resulting in a very rigid and non-compliant structure [49, 75] that changes minimally (~1.4%) with

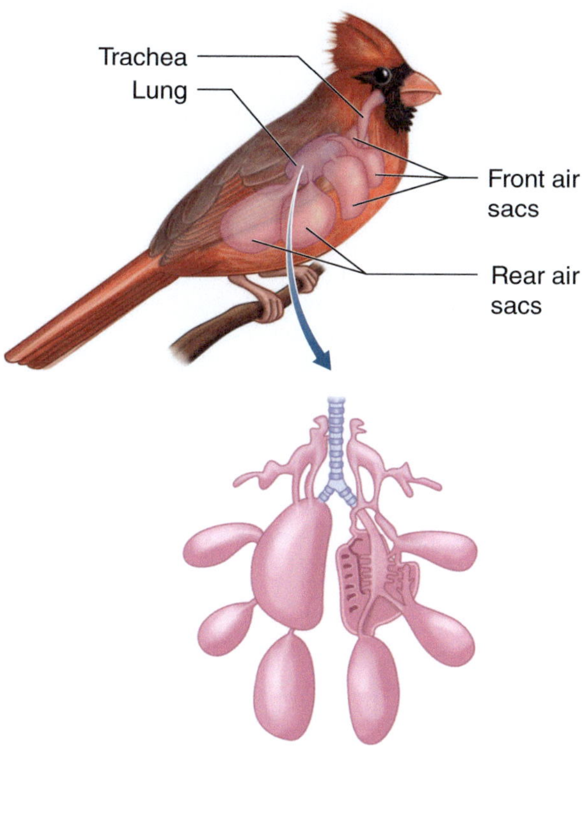

Fig. 6.4 The avian respiratory system is unique in that the respiratory surface (paired lungs/parabronchi) is uncoupled from the ventilatory aspect (air sacs). Furthermore, the avian lung exhibits cross-current gas exchange, meaning that airflow is one-way through the lung

each breath [114]. In contrast, the air sacs are highly compliant and act similar to bellows [102]. Birds have multiple cranial and caudal air sacs that vary in size, location, and connections [115, 116], but they do not act as a respiratory surface.

The lungs are continuously ventilated from back to front, and require two inspiratory and expiratory cycles for a given volume of air to move through the system [115]. Active expiration occurs in birds, unlike passive expiration observed in resting mammals [117]. Breathing occurs through chest cavity expansions and reductions via inspiratory and expiratory muscles. During inspiration, air moves from the outside environment into the caudal air sacs at the same time as air moves across the lungs into the cranial air sacs [11, 49]. On expiration, air from the cranial air sacs exits through the trachea while air from the caudal air sacs moves through the lung [115]. Caudal air sacs therefore have a higher O_2 concentration compared to the cranial air sacs, which have a higher CO_2 concentration [108]. This style of breathing results in no dead space ventilation, unlike in the mammalian lung.

High-Altitude Hypoxia

Their efficient respiratory system allows birds to conduct high-intensity exercise in hypoxic environments without prior acclimatization, a feat that would be extremely difficult for other mammals [106, 118, 119]. Many bird species experience hypobaric hypoxia around the globe, either as permanent high-altitude residents (such as the Andean goose [*Chloephaga melanoptera*] found in the Andean Altiplano), through vertical migration (observed in the giant hummingbird [*Patagona gigas*] and bar-headed goose [*Anser indicus*] [120]), or briefly during migratory flights (such as the great reed warbler [*Acrocephalus arundinaceus*] [121]; [122]). Although they are able to tolerate greater degrees of hypoxia compared to mammals, birds still exhibit ventilatory responses to hypoxia. Bar-headed geese and some high-altitude Andean duck species have greater ventilatory responses to hypoxia compared to low-altitude species, with contributions of both tidal volume and breathing frequency [123–126]. Bar-headed geese have reduced CO_2 sensitivity compared to other geese species, allowing for further increases in ventilation with reduced restraint of respiratory hypocapnia/alkalosis on ventilation [126, 127] and blunted hypocapnic cerebral vasoconstriction [128]. This reduced CO_2 sensitivity is important during flight to maintain O_2 uptake, when ventilation is high, and O_2 movement to the brain and heart.

In contrast, Andean geese have a blunted hypoxic ventilatory response but high pulmonary O_2 extraction [125], which is supported by significant modifications to lung structure [129]. The Andean goose lung has highly vascularized infundibula (the structures from which the air capillaries arise), increasing the respiratory surface area and volume of pulmonary capillary blood available for gas exchange [129]. This modification allows them to have the highest mass-specific respiratory surface area reported in birds to date [129]. The blood–gas barrier is also thicker in Andean geese compared to other birds, which may aid in preventing structural failure during flights at high altitude, where heart rate and cardiac output would be elevated [129]. How these lung structures compare to Bar-headed geese is unknown, but many other highland-resident duck species exhibit larger mass-specific lung volumes compared to lowland species, suggesting that Bar-headed geese may also have changes in lung structure [130].

Breathing is energetically expensive, with elastic work increasing exponentially with tidal volume, but only linearly increasing with breathing frequency [70]. As noted above, many high-altitude bird species increase tidal volume in response to hypoxia, suggesting that they may reduce the cost of breathing through increases in compliance and/or increasing the size of the respiratory system relative to body size [131]. Andean geese have disproportionately larger respiratory volumes compared to bar-headed geese, allowing them to breathe deeply for the same energetic cost as geese of the same size [131]. In contrast, many high-altitude Andean duck species have more compliant respiratory systems compared to lowland sister taxa [132], although these changes in compliance did not significantly reduce the work of breathing [132].

Diving

Diving is common in many bird species and the challenges previously discussed with deep diving and the mammalian lung are applicable to the avian respiratory system, despite the stiff avian lung. Variation in dive depth is observed across penguin species, allowing for comparison of adaptations in lung physiology between deep-diving penguins, such as emperor penguins (*Aptenodytes forsteri*) (diving up to 400 m deep) [133–136], and shallow divers, such as Adélie penguins (*Pygoscelis adeliae*) (diving between 10 and 40 m deep) [137–139]. As with diving mammals, mass-specific lung volumes are smaller in deep-diving penguins compared to shallow-diving species [140–142]. Smaller volumes allow for lower air capillary and parabronchial volumes, which would protect against barotrauma during deep dives [142]. Additionally, deep-diving penguins have greater lung compliance, up to six times greater than shallow divers, suggesting that the lung may compress and reduce volume at deep-dive depths to further protect against barotrauma [142]. The blood–gas barrier is also thicker in penguins compared to other bird species, which would aid in preventing the lungs from collapsing under high hydrostatic pressures [140, 143]. Air capillaries are very unlikely to collapse at deep-dive depths, due to the difficulty of re-expanding an area with such a small diameter and radius of curvature [144, 145].

Penguins and some diving ducks also exhibit modifications in their skeleton to support breathing upon surfacing and submergence. Diving birds have elongated ribs, ribcage, and sternum compared to walking species, suggesting that added skeletal support may be required for breathing during resurfacing, as inspiration occurs against the pressure of water against the body [146]. Air sac walls are also thicker in diving birds, which would aid in preventing collapse during dives [142, 147]. Diving birds also exhibit variation in breathing strategy before diving, with penguins inspiring before dives [148, 149], while ducks such as lesser scaups (*Aythya affinis*) exhale before diving [150]. Why there is variation in breathing strategy among diving birds has not been well investigated, but it may be associated with dive depth. In free-diving penguins, inhalation before diving results in diving air volumes that are 30–50% greater than allometrically predicted respiratory volumes [148, 149].

Exercise and High Temperatures

Ostriches (*Struthio camelus*) and other ratites (large, flightless birds of the Southern Hemisphere) are known for their high exercise capacity and ability to endure high thermal stress. Volant birds may experience heat stress from exercise (i.e. flying), but can use adiabatic cooling (i.e. flying at higher altitudes) and convective heat loss during flight [141]. Ostriches presumably experience heat stress during exercise, as they can sustain running speeds of up to 90 km/h, but are also known to experience heat stress when at rest. To support their high running speeds, ostriches have an extensive respiratory surface area and a thick blood–gas barrier (comparable to that of Humboldt penguins [*Spheniscus humboldti*] [140]). Although counter-intuitive, a thick blood–gas barrier supports the high volumes of blood that would pass through the lungs during exercise, preventing damage to the pulmonary vasculature [141].

As ratites are unable to easily seek protection from the sun, like other small birds, they have evolved adaptations to prevent overheating. In addition to maintaining a lower body temperature compared to other birds (38–40 °C compared to 40–42 °C) [141, 151, 152], ostriches and emus (*Dromaius novaehollandiae*) are able to maintain resting levels of arterial PCO_2 and pH after panting for 6 h when exposed to 56 °C [153–155]. Birds typically exhibit panting when exposed to heat stress, leading to respiratory alkalosis [156, 157]. It is suggested that in panting ostriches the increased airflow from the caudal air sac results in a large proportion of the air bypassing the lungs and instead moving back towards the trachea [141]. Maina and Nathaniel [141] suggest that there may be an expiratory aerodynamic valving mechanism that facilitates this process. As the gas exchange surface is bypassed, the air sacs therefore provide evaporative cooling to the animal [141]. Increases in the homogeneity of blood flow in the lungs have also been observed during panting compared to resting conditions in ostriches [154], supporting the changes in lung ventilation.

Conclusion

Respiratory organs have been challenged by external environments and species requirements, resulting in a variety of adaptations that sustain O_2 uptake. The transition to land challenged the appearance of respiratory organs (evaginated versus invaginated), but they maintained their common set of characteristics (free movement of blood in a large capillary network, thin and moist gas exchange surface, and constant renewal of O_2-rich media to provide O_2 and remove CO_2). Here, we have highlighted many similar responses of respiratory organs to environmental extremes throughout vertebrate taxa. High-endurance species have a greater reliance on reinforced respiratory structures to endure high blood flows. Animals inhabiting hypoxic environments (aquatic or terrestrial) exhibit more effective breathing patterns (slower, deeper breaths) and have altered perfusion of respiratory organs to match their environment. For many deep-diving mammals and birds, they have smaller lung volumes, more compliant lungs to support compression, and reinforced conducting airways compared to shallow-diving species. All of these responses highlight the ability of respiratory structures to respond to environmental extremes and ultimately maintain O_2 uptake.

References

1. Carvalho O, Gonçalves C. Comparative physiology of the respiratory system in the animal kingdom. Open Biol J. 2011;4:35–46.
2. Grunwald DJ. A Fin-de-Siecle achievement: charting new waters in vertebrate biology. Science. 1996;274:1634–5.
3. Maina JN. Comparative respiratory physiology: the fundamental mechanisms and the functional designs of the gas exchangers. Open Access Anim Physiol. 2014;53
4. Maina JN. Fundamental structural aspects and features in the bioengineering of the gas exchangers: comparative perspectives. Cell Biol: Adv Anat Embryol; 2002. p. 163.
5. Milsom WK, Gilmour KM, Perry S, Gargaglioni LH, Hedrick MS, Kinkead R, Wang T. Control of breathing in ectothermic vertebrates. Compr Physiol. 2022; https://doi.org/10.1002/cphy.c210041.
6. Borowiec BG, Leonard EM. The hypoxic ventilatory response and oxygen sensing in fishes. Encycl Fish Physiol. 2024:107–18.
7. Powell FL, Milsom WK, Mitchell GS. Time domains of the hypoxic ventilatory response. Respir Physiol. 1998;112:123–34.
8. Porteus C, Hedrick MS, Hicks JW, Wang T, Milsom WK. Time domains of the hypoxic ventilatory response in ectothermic vertebrates. J Comp Physiol B Biochem Syst Environ Physiol. 2011;181:311–33.
9. Milsom WK. Adaptive trends in respiratory control: a comparative perspective. Am J Physiol Regul Integr Comp Physiol. 2010; https://doi.org/10.1152/ajpregu.00069.2010.
10. Evans DH, Piermarini PM, Choe KP. The multifunctional fish gill: dominant site of gas exchange, osmoregulation, acid-base regulation, and excretion of nitrogenous waste. Physiol Rev. 2005;85:97–177.
11. Maina JN. Comparative respiratory morphology: themes and principles in the design and construction of the gas exchangers. Anat Rec. 2000;261:25.
12. Olson K. Gill circulation: regulation of perfusion distribution and metabolism of regulatory molecules. J Exp Zool. 2002;293:320–35.
13. Perry SF. The chloride cell: structure and function in the gills of freshwater fishes. Annu Rev Physiol. 1997;59:325–47.
14. Moyle PB, Cech JJ (2004) Respiration. Fishes An Introd to Ichthyol. https://doi.org/10.2307/1447679.

15. Perry SF, Jonz MG, Gilmour KM. Chapter 5. Oxygen sensing and the hypoxic ventilatory response. In: Fish Physiol; 2009. p. 193–253.
16. Bushnell PG, Brill RW. Responses of swimming skipjack (Katsuwonus pelamis) and yellowfin (Thunnus albacares) tunas to acute hypoxia, and a model of their cardiorespiratory function. Physiol Zool. 1991;64:787–811.
17. Winemiller KO. Development of dermal lip protuberances for aquatic surface respiration in South American characid fishes. Copeia. 1989;1989:382.
18. Olson KR, Dewar H, Graham JB, Brill RW. Vascular anatomy of the gills in a high energy demand teleost, the skipjack tuna (Katsuwonus pelamis). J Exp Zool Part A Comp Exp Biol. 2003;297:17–31.
19. Muir BS, Hughes GM. Gill dimensions for three species of tunny. J Exp Biol. 1969;51:271–85.
20. Muir BS, Brown CE. Effects of blood pathway on the blood-pressure drop in fish gills, with special reference to tunas. J Fish Res Board Canada. 1971;28:947–55.
21. Muir BS, Kendall JI. Structural modifications in the gills of tunas and some other oceanic fishes. Copeia. 1968;1968:388.
22. Gray IE. Comparative study of the gill area of marine fishes. Biol Bull. 1954;107.
23. Long NP, Farina SC. Enormous gill chambers of deep-sea coffinfishes (Lophiiformes: Chaunacidae) support unique ventilatory specialisations such as breath holding and extreme inflation. J Fish Biol. 2019;95:502–9.
24. Randall DJ, Baumgarten D, Malyusz M. The relationship between gas and ion transfer across the gills of fishes. Comp Biochem Physiol Part A Physiol. 1972;41:629–37.
25. Nilsson GE. Gill remodeling in fish—a new fashion or an ancient secret? J Exp Biol. 2007;210:2403–9.
26. Sollid J, De Angelis P, Gundersen K, Nilsson GE. Hypoxia induces adaptive and reversible gross morphological changes in crucian carp gills. J Exp Biol. 2003;206:3667–73.
27. McDonald DG, McMahon BR. Respiratory development in Arctic char Salvelinus alpinus under conditions of normoxia and chronic hypoxia. Can J Zool. 1977;55:1461–7.
28. Matey V, Iftikar FI, de Boeck G, Scott GR, Sloman KA, Almeida-Val VMF, Val AL, Wood CM. Gill morphology and acute hypoxia: responses of mitochondria-rich, pavement, and mucous cells in the Amazonian oscar (Astronotus ocellatus) and the rainbow trout (Oncorhynchus mykiss), two species with very different approaches to the osmo-respiratory com. Can J Zool. 2011;89:307–24.
29. Borowiec BG, Darcy KL, Gillette DM, Scott GR. Distinct physiological strategies are used to cope with constant hypoxia and intermittent hypoxia in killifish (Fundulus heteroclitus). J Exp Biol. 2015;218:1198–211.
30. Chasiotis H, Kolosov D, Bui P, Kelly SP. Tight junctions, tight junction proteins and paracellular permeability across the gill epithelium of fishes: a review. Respir Physiol Neurobiol. 2012;184:269–81.
31. Rankin JC, Tuurala H. Gills of Antarctic fish. Comp Biochem Physiol Part A Mol Integr Physiol. 1998;119:149–63.
32. Ruud JT. Vertebrates without erythrocytes and blood pigment. Nature. 1954;173:848–50.
33. Holeton GF. Oxygen uptake and circulation by a hemoglobinless antarctic fish (Chaenocephalus aceratus Lonnberg) compared with three red-blooded Antartic fish. Comp Biochem Physiol. 1970;34:457–71.
34. Scott GR, Wood CM, Sloman KA, Iftikar FI, De Boeck G, Almeida-Val VMF, Val AL. Respiratory responses to progressive hypoxia in the Amazonian oscar, Astronotus ocellatus. Respir Physiol Neurobiol. 2008;162:109–16.
35. Wood CM, Iftikar FI, Scott GR, De Boeck G, Sloman KA, Matey V, Domingos FXV, Duarte RM, Almeida-Val VMF, Val AL. Regulation of gill transcellular permeability and renal function during acute hypoxia in the Amazonian oscar (Astronotus ocellatus): new angles to the osmorespiratory compromise. J Exp Biol. 2009;212:1949–64.

36. Leite CAC, Florindo LH, Kalinin AL, Milsom WK, Rantin FT. Gill chemoreceptors and cardio-respiratory reflexes in the neotropical teleost pacu, Piaractus mesopotamicus. J Comp Physiol A Neuroethol Sensory, Neural, Behav Physiol. 2007;193:1001–11.
37. Oliveira RD, Lopes JM, Sanches JR, Kalinin AL, Glass ML, Rantin FT. Cardiorespiratory responses of the facultative air-breathing fish jeju, Hoplerythrinus unitaeniatus (Teleostei, Erythrinidae), exposed to graded ambient hypoxia. Comp Biochem Physiol A Mol Integr Physiol. 2004;139:479–85.
38. De Moraes MFPG, Höller S, Da Costa OTF, Glass ML, Fernandes MN, Perry SF. Morphometric comparison of the respiratory organs in the South American lungfish Lepidosiren paradoxa (Dipnoi). Physiol Biochem Zool. 2005;78:546–59.
39. Shelton G. The regulation of breathing. Fish Physiol. 1970;4:293–359.
40. Burggren WW, Johansen K. Circulation and respiration in lungfishes (dipnoi). J Morphol. 1986;190:217–36.
41. Hughes GM. Species variation in gas exchange. Proc R Soc B Biol Sci. 1966;59:494–500.
42. Val AL. Fishes of the Amazon: diversity and beyond. An Acad Bras Cienc. 2019;91:e20190260.
43. Little C. The terrestrial invasion: an ecophysiological approach to the origins of land animals. Terr invasion an Ecophysiol approach to Orig L Anim. 1990; https://doi.org/10.1016/0169-5347(91)90095-f.
44. Cupello C, Hirasawa T, Tatsumi N, et al. Lung evolution in vertebrates and the water-to-land transition. Elife. 2022; https://doi.org/10.7554/ELIFE.77156.
45. Riddell EA, Burger IJ, Muñoz MM, Weaver SJ, Womack MC. Amphibians exhibit extremely high hydric costs of respiration. Integr Comp Biol. 2024; https://doi.org/10.1093/icb/icae053.
46. Bentley PJ, Yorio T. Evaporative water loss in anuran amphibia: a comparative study. Comp Biochem Physiol Part A Physiol. 1979;62:1005–9.
47. Burggren W, Moallf R. "Active" regulation of cutaneous exchange by capillary recruitment in amphibians: experimental evidence and a revised model for skin respiration. Respir Physiol. 1984;55:379–92.
48. Burggren WW, Vitalis TZ. The interplay of cutaneous water loss, gas exchange and blood flow in the toad, Bufo woodhousei: adaptations in a terrestrially adapted amphibian. J Exp Biol. 2005;208:105–12.
49. Duncker HR. Vertebrate lungs: structure, topography and mechanics. A comparative perspective of the progressive integration of respiratory system, locomotor apparatus and ontogenetic development. Respir Physiol Neurobiol. 2004;144:111–24.
50. Carrier DR, Wake MH. Mechanism of lung ventilation in the caecilian Dermophis mexicanus. J Morphol. 1995;226:289–95.
51. Maina JN, Maloiy GMO. A scanning and transmission electron microscopic study of the lung of a caecilian Boulengerula taitanus. J Zool. 1988;215:739–51.
52. Gatz RN, Crawford EC, Piiper J. Respiratory properties of the blood of a lungless and gill-less salamander, Desmognathus fuscus. Respir Physiol. 1974;20:33–41.
53. Full RJ, Anderson BD, Finnerty CM, Feder ME. Exercising with and without lungs: I. The effects of metabolic cost, maximal oxygen transport and body size on terrestrial locomotion in salamander species. J Exp Biol. 1988;138:471–85.
54. Czopek J. The vascularization of the respiratory surfaces of some Salientia. Zool Pol. 1955;6:101–34.
55. Czopek J. Vascularization of respiratory surfaces in some caudata. Copeia. 1962;1962:576.
56. Tenney SM, Tenney JB. Quantitative morphology of cold-blooded lungs: amphibia and reptilia. Respir Physiol. 1970;9:197–215.
57. Withers PC, Hedrick MS, Drewes RC, Hillman SS. Pulmonary compliance and lung volume are related to terrestriality in Anuran Amphibians. Physiol Biochem Zool. 2014;87:374–83.
58. Burggren W, Mwalukoma A. Respiration during chronic hypoxia and hyperoxia in larval and adult bullfrogs (Rana catesbeiana). I. Morphological responses of lungs, skin and gills. J Exp Biol. 1983;105:191–203.

59. Noble GK, Pope CH. The adaptive modifications of the arboreal tadpoles of Hoplophryne and the torrent tadpoles of Staurois. Bull Am Museum Nat Hist. 1929;58:291.
60. Howell BJ. Acid-base balance in transition from water breathing to air breathing. Fed Proc. 1970;29:1130–4.
61. Maina JN. Structure, function and evolution of the gas exchangers: comparative perspectives. J Anat. 2002;201:281–304.
62. Skovgaard N, Abe AS, Andrade DV, Wang T. Hypoxic pulmonary vasoconstriction in reptiles: a comparative study of four species with different lung structures and pulmonary blood pressures. Am J Physiol Regul Integr Comp Physiol. 2005; https://doi.org/10.1152/ajpregu.00200.2005.
63. Perry SF. Reptilian lungs. Functional anatomy and evolution. Adv Anat Embryol Cell Biol. 1983;79:1–81.
64. Fleetwood JN, Munnell JF. Morphology of the airways and lung parenchyma in hatchlings of the loggerhead sea turtle, Caretta caretta. J Morphol. 1996;227:289–304.
65. Bickler PE, Buck LT. Hypoxia tolerance in reptiles, amphibians, and fishes: life with variable oxygen availability. Annu Rev Physiol. 2007;69:145–70.
66. Tenney SM, Bartlett D, Farber JP, Remmers JE. Mechanics of the respiratory cycle in the green turtle (Chelonia mydas). Respir Physiol. 1974;22:361–8.
67. Gans C, Clark B. Studies on ventilation of Caiman crocodilus (crocodilia: Reptilia). Respir Physiol. 1976;26:285–301.
68. Lutcavage ME, Bushnell PG, Jones DR. Oxygen stores and aerobic metabolism in the leatherback sea turtle. Can J Zool. 1992;70:348–51.
69. Lutcavage ME, Lutz PL, Baier H. Respiratory mechanics of the loggerhead sea turtle, Caretta caretta. Respir Physiol. 1989;76:13–24.
70. Vitalis TZ, Milsom WK. Pulmonary mechanics and the work of breathing in the semi-aquatic turtle, Pseudemys scripta. J Exp Biol. 1986;125:137–55.
71. Gatz RN, Glass ML, Wood SC. Pulmonary function of the green sea turtle, Chelonia mydas. J Appl Physiol. 1987;62:459–63.
72. Hochscheid S, McMahon CR, Bradshaw CJA, Maffucci F, Bentivegna F, Hays GC. Allometric scaling of lung volume and its consequences for marine turtle diving performance. Comp Biochem Physiol A Mol Integr Physiol. 2007;148:360–7.
73. Hicks JW, Farmer CG. Gas exchange potential in reptilian lungs: implications for the dinosaur-avian connection. Respir Physiol. 1999;117:73–83.
74. Duncker HR. The emergence of macroscopic complexity: an outline of the history of the respiratory apparatus of vertebrates from diffusion to language production. Zoology. 2001;103:240–59.
75. West JB, Watson RR, Fu Z. The honeycomb-like structure of the bird lung allows a uniquely thin blood-gas barrier. Respir Physiol Neurobiol. 2006;152:115–8.
76. Ivy CM, Scott GR. Control of breathing and ventilatory acclimatization to hypoxia in deer mice native to high altitudes. Acta Physiol. 2017;221:266–82.
77. Pichon A, Zhenzhong B, Marchant D, Jin G, Voituron N, Haixia Y, Favret F, Richalet J-P, Ge R-L. Cardiac adaptation to high altitude in the plateau pika (Ochotona curzoniae). Physiol Rep. 2013;1:e00032.
78. Ge RL, Kubo K, Kobayashi T, Sekiguchi M, Honda T. Blunted hypoxic pulmonary vasoconstrictive response in the rodent Ochotona curzoniae (pika) at high altitude. Am J Physiol. 1998;274:H1792–9.
79. Durmowicz AG, Hofmeister S, Kadyraliev TK, Aldashev AA, Stenmark KR. Functional and structural adaptation of the yak pulmonary circulation to residence at high altitude. J Appl Physiol. 1993;74:2276–85.
80. Anand IS, Harris E, Ferrari R, Pearce P, Harris P. Pulmonary haemodynamics of the yak, cattle, and cross breeds at high altitude. Thorax. 1986;41:696–700.
81. Harris P, Heath D, Smith P, Williams DR, Ramirez A, Krüger H, Jones DM. Pulmonary circulation of llama at high and low altitudes. Thorax. 1982;37:38–45.

82. Ishizaki T, Sakai A, Koizumi T, Ruan Z, Wang ZG. Blunted effect of the Kv channel inhibitor on pulmonary circulation in Tibetan sheep: a model for studying hypoxia and pulmonary artery pressure regulation. Respirology. 2004;9:125–9.
83. Piscitelli MA, McLellan WA, Rommel SA, Blum JE, Barco SG, Ann Pabst D. Lung size and thoracic morphology in shallow- and deep-diving cetaceans. J Morphol. 2010;271:654–73.
84. Ridgway SH, Howard R. Dolphin lung collapse and intramuscular circulation during free diving: evidence from nitrogen washout. Science. 1979;206:1182–3.
85. Fahlman A, Moore MJ, Garcia-Parraga D. Respiratory function and mechanics in pinnipeds and cetaceans. J Exp Biol. 2017;220:1761–73.
86. Scholander PF. Experimental investigations on the respiratory function in diving mammals and birds. Hvalrad Skr. 1940:1–131.
87. Kooyman GL. Respiratory adaptations in marine mammals. Integr Comp Biol. 1973;13:457–68.
88. Leith DE. Adaptations to deep breath-hold diving: respiratory and circulatory mechanics. Undersea Biomed Res. 1989;16:345–54.
89. Piscitelli MA, Raverty SA, Lillie MA, Shadwick RE. A review of cetacean lung morphology and mechanics. J Morphol. 2013;274:1425–40.
90. Fahlman A, Loring SH, Johnson SP, Haulena M, Trites AW, Fravel VA, van Bonn WG. Inflation and deflation pressure-volume loops in anesthetized pinnipeds confirms compliant chest and lungs. Front Physiol. 2014; https://doi.org/10.3389/fphys.2014.00433.
91. Leith DE. Comparative mammalian respiratory mechanics. Dis: Am Rev Respir; 1983. p. 128.
92. Kooyman GL, Sinnett EE. Pulmonary shunts in harbor seals and sea lions during simulated dives to depth. Physiol Zool. 1982;55:105–11.
93. Baković D, Valic Z, Eterović D, Vuković I, Obad A, Marinović-Terzić I, Dujić Ž. Spleen volume and blood flow response to repeated breath-hold apneas. J Appl Physiol. 2003;95:1460–6.
94. Kooyman GL. Physiology without restraint in diving mammals. Mar Mammal Sci. 1985;1:166–78.
95. Butler PJ. Exercise in birds. J Exp Biol. 1991;160:233–62.
96. Maina JN, Thomas SP, Hyde DM. A morphometric study of the lungs of different sized bats: correlations between structure and function of the chiropteran lung. Philos Trans R Soc Lond B Biol Sci. 1991;333:31–50.
97. Maina JN, King AS. The structural functional correlation in the design of the bat lung. A morphometric study. J Exp Biol. 1984;111:43–63.
98. Maina JN. What it takes to fly: the structural and functional respiratory refinements in birds and bats. J Exp Biol. 2000;203:3045–64.
99. Hartman F. Some flight mechanisms of bats. Ohio J Sci. 1963;63:59–65.
100. Jürgens KD, Bartels H, Bartels R. Blood oxygen transport and organ weights of small bats and small non-flying mammals. Respir Physiol. 1981;45:243–60.
101. Mathieu-Costello O, Szewczak JM, Logemann RB, Agey PJ. Geometry of blood-tissue exchange in bat flight muscle compared with bat hindlimb and rat soleus muscle. Am J Physiol Regul Integr Comp Physiol. 1992; https://doi.org/10.1152/ajpregu.1992.262.6.r955.
102. Maina JN. The biology of the avian respiratory system: evolution, development, structure and function. Biol Avian Respir Syst Evol Dev Struct Funct. 2017; https://doi.org/10.1007/978-3-319-44153-5.
103. Lasiewski RC, Dawson WR. A re-examination of the relation between standard metabolic rate and body weight in birds. Condor. 1967;69:13–23.
104. Aschoff J, Pohl H. Rhythmic variations in energy metabolism. Fed Proc. 1970;29:1541–52.
105. Hunter P. The nature of flight. The molecules and mechanics of flight in animals. EMBO Rep. 2007;8:811–3.
106. Lasiewski RC. Respiratory function in birds. In: Avian Biol; 1972. p. 287–342.
107. Perry SF. Functional morphology of the lungs of the Nile crocodile, Crocodylus niloticus: non-respiratory parameters. J Exp Biol. 1988;134:99–117.
108. Scheid P. Respiration and control of breathing. In: Avian Biol; 1982. p. 405–53.

109. Scott GR. Elevated performance: the unique physiology of birds that fly at high altitudes. J Exp Biol. 2011;214:2455–62.
110. Milsom WK, Hawkes LA, Meir JU, Scott GR, Frappell PB. Point: high altitude is for the birds! J Appl Physiol. 2011;111:1514–5.
111. Powell FL, Hastings RH, Mazzone RW. Pulmonary vascular resistance during unilateral pulmonary arterial occlusion in ducks. Am J Physiol Regul Integr Comp Physiol. 1985; https://doi.org/10.1152/ajpregu.1985.249.1.r39.
112. West JB. Comparative physiology of the pulmonary blood-gas barrier: the unique avian solution. Am J Physiol Regul Integr Comp Physiol. 2009; https://doi.org/10.1152/ajpregu.00459.2009.
113. Watson RR, Fu Z, West JB. Minimal distensibility of pulmonary capillaries in avian lungs compared with mammalian lungs. Respir Physiol Neurobiol. 2008;160:208–14.
114. Jones JH, Effmann EL, Schmidt-Nielsen K. Lung volume changes during respiration in ducks. Respir Physiol. 1985;59:15–25.
115. Maina JN. Perspectives on the structure and function of the avian respiratory system: functional efficiency built on structural complexity. Front Anim Sci. 2022; https://doi.org/10.3389/fanim.2022.851574.
116. King AS. Structural and functional aspects of the avian lungs and air sacs. Int Rev Gen Exp Zool. 1966;2:171–267.
117. Codd JR, Boggs DF, Perry SF, Carrier DR. Activity of three muscles associated with the uncinate processes of the giant Canada goose Branta canadensis maximus. J Exp Biol. 2005;208:849–57.
118. Tucker VA. Respiratory physiology of house sparrows in relation to high-altitude flight. J Exp Biol. 1968;48:55–66.
119. Maina JN. Scanning electron microscope study of the spatial organization of the air and blood conducting components of the avian lung (Gallus Gallus variant domesticus). Anat Rec. 1988;222:145–53.
120. Williamson JL, Witt CC. Elevational niche-shift migration: why the degree of elevational change matters for the ecology, evolution, and physiology of migratory birds. Ornithology. 2021; https://doi.org/10.1093/ORNITHOLOGY/UKAA087.
121. Sjöberg S, Malmiga G, Nord A, et al. Extreme altitudes during diurnal flights in a nocturnal songbird migrant. Science. 2021;372:646–8.
122. Ivy CM, Williamson JL. On the physiology of high-altitude flight and altitudinal migration in birds. Integr Comp Biol. 2024.
123. Black CP, Tenney SM. Oxygen transport during progressive hypoxia in high-altitude and sea-level waterfowl. Respir Physiol. 1980;39:217–39.
124. Lague SL, Chua B, Farrell AP, Wang Y, Milsom WK. Altitude matters: differences in cardiovascular and respiratory responses to hypoxia in bar-headed geese reared at high and low altitudes. J Exp Biol. 2016;219:1974–84.
125. Lague SL, Chua B, Alza L, Scott GR, Frappell PB, Zhong Y, Farrell AP, McCracken KG, Wang Y, Milsom WK. Divergent respiratory and cardiovascular responses to hypoxia in bar-headed geese and Andean birds. J Exp Biol. 2017;220:4186–94.
126. Scott GR, Milsom WK. Control of breathing and adaptation to high altitude in the bar-headed goose. AJP Regul Integr Comp Physiol. 2007;293:R379–91.
127. Scott GR, Milsom WK. Control of breathing in birds: implications for high altitude flight. In: Glass ML, Wood SC, editors. Cardio-respiratory Control Vertebr. Comp. Evol. Asp. Berlin: Springer; 2009. p. 429–88.
128. Faraci FM, Fedde MR. Regional circulatory responses to hypocapnia and hypercapnia in bar-headed geese. Am J Physiol Regul Integr Comp Physiol. 1986; https://doi.org/10.1152/ajpregu.1986.250.3.r499.
129. Maina JN, McCracken KG, Chua B, York JM, Milsom WK. Morphological and morphometric specializations of the lung of the Andean goose, Chloephaga melanoptera: a lifelong high-altitude resident. PLoS One. 2017;12:e0174395.

130. Bakkeren C, Smith E, York JM, Chua B, McCracken KG, Milsom WK. A morphometric analysis of the lungs of high-altitude ducks and geese. J Anat. 2020;237:188–96.
131. York JM, Scadeng M, McCracken KG, Milsom WK. Respiratory mechanics and morphology of Tibetan and Andean high-altitude geese with divergent life histories. J Exp Biol. 2018; https://doi.org/10.1242/jeb.170738.
132. York JM, Chua BA, Ivy CM, et al. Respiratory mechanics of eleven avian species resident at high and low altitude. J Exp Biol. 2017;220:1079–89.
133. Kirkwood R, Robertson G. Seasonal change in the foraging ecology of emperor penguins on the Mawson Coast, Antarctica. Mar Ecol Prog Ser. 1997;156:205–23.
134. Kooyman GL, Kooyman TG. Diving behavior of emperor penguins nurturing chicks at Coulman Island, Antarctica. Condor. 1995;97:536–49.
135. Rodary D, Bonneau W, Le Maho Y, Bost CA. Benthic diving in male emperor penguins Aptenodytes forsteri foraging in winter. Mar Ecol Prog Ser. 2000;207:171–81.
136. Wienecke B, Robertson G, Kirkwood R, Lawton K. Extreme dives by free-ranging emperor penguins. Polar Biol. 2007;30:133–42.
137. Chappell MA, Shoemaker VH, Janes DN, Bucher TL, Maloney SK. Diving behavior during foraging in breeding Adelie penguins. Ecology. 1993;74:1204–15.
138. Norman FI, Ward SJ. Foraging group size and dive duration of Adelie penguins Pygoscelis adeliae at sea off Hop Island, Rauer Group, East Antarctica. Mar Ornithol. 1993;21:37–47.
139. Watanuki Y, Kato A, Naito Y, Robertson G, Robinson S. Diving and foraging behaviour of Adelie penguins in areas with and without fast sea-ice. Polar Biol. 1997;17:296–304.
140. Maina JN, King AS. A morphometric study of the lung of a Humboldt penguin (Sphenicus humboldti). Anat Histol Embryol. 1987;16.
141. Maina JN, Nathaniel C. A qualitative and quantitative study of the lung of an ostrich, Struthio camelus. J Exp Biol. 2001;204:2313–30.
142. Ponganis PJ, St Leger J, Scadeng M. Penguin lungs and air sacs: implications for baroprotection, oxygen stores and buoyancy. J Exp Biol. 2015;218:720–30.
143. Welsch U, Aschauer B. Ultrastructural observations on the lung of the emperor penguin (Aptenodytes forsten). Cell Tissue Res. 1986;243:137–44.
144. Duncker HR. Structure of avian lungs. Respir Physiol. 1972;14:44–63.
145. Duncker HR. Structure of the avian respiratory tract. Respir Physiol. 1974;22:1–19.
146. Tickle PG, Ennos AR, Lennox LE, Perry SF, Codd JR. Functional significance of the uncinate processes in birds. J Exp Biol. 2007;210:3955–61.
147. Jaensch S. Inspirational evolution: the avian lower respiratory tract. 2015;23:1–11.
148. Sato K, Naito Y, Kato A, Niizuma Y, Watanuki T, Sharrassin JB, Bost C-A, Handrich Y, Le Maho Y. Buoyancy and maximal diving depth in penguins do they control inhaling air volume. J Exp Biol. 2002;205:1189–97.
149. Sato K, Shiomi K, Marshall G, Kooyman GL, Ponganis PJ. Stroke rates and diving air volumes of emperor penguins: implications for dive performance. J Exp Biol. 2011;214:2854–63.
150. Lasiewski RC, Calder WA. A preliminary allometric analysis of respiratory variables in resting birds. Respir Physiol. 1971;11:152–66.
151. Bligh J, Hartley TC. the deep body temperature of an unrestrained ostrich Struthio camelus recorded continuously by a radio-telemetric technique. Ibis (Lond 1859). 1965;107:104–5.
152. Crawford EC, Schmidt-Nielsen K. Temperature regulation and evaporative cooling in the ostrich. Am J Physiol. 1967;212:347–53.
153. Schmidt-Nielsen K, Kanwisher J, Lasiewski RC, Cohn JE, Bretz WL. Temperature regulation and respiration in the ostrich. Condor. 1969;71:341–52.
154. Jones JH. Pulmonary blood flow distribution in panting ostriches. J Appl Physiol Respir Environ Exerc Physiol. 1982;53:1411–7.
155. Jones JH, Grubb B, Schmidt-Nielsen K. Panting in the emu causes arterialhypoxemia. Respir Physiol Neurobiol. 1983;54:189–95.

156. Calder WA, Schmidt-Nielsen K. Evaporative cooling and respiratory alkalosis in the pigeon. Proc Natl Acad Sci U S A. 1966;55:750–6.
157. Calder WA, Schmidt-Nielsen K. Panting and blood carbon dioxide in birds. Am J Physiol. 1968;215:477–82.

Chapter 7
Physiology and Pathophysiology of the Lungs in the Fetus, Newborn, and Young Child

Weston T. Powell and Deborah R. Liptzin

Introduction

The transition from the intrauterine environment to the extrauterine environment is one of the most dramatic physiologic changes that a human experiences. Over the course of a few breaths, the lung changes from a primarily secretory organ to a primarily absorptive organ, the epithelium transitions from a liquid–liquid interface to an air–liquid interface, and responsibility for gas exchange shifts from the placenta to the lungs, which now receive significantly more blood flow. The normal neonatal lung demonstrates bronchovascular bundles containing the airways and the pulmonary arteries, complex alveoli comprised primarily of flat type I alveolar epithelial cells interspersed with plump type II alveolar epithelial cells, and an interstitium comprised primarily of capillaries for rapid gas exchange and pulmonary veins (Fig. 7.1: normal lung at term). Somehow all these processes progress normally in every delivered healthy baby. The infant faces a series of physiologic challenges through the neonatal period as the infant adjusts to the transition from the intrauterine environment to the extrauterine environment. For example, while the very compliant chest wall eases passage through the birth canal, it impairs pulmonary mechanics in the postnatal period. In this chapter, we discuss these normal processes as well as the means by which things go wrong, including transient

Images and descriptions courtesy of Gail H Deutsch MD Department of Laboratory Medicine and Pathology, University of Washington, Seattle, WA. The authors would like to acknowledge her generous contributions.

W. T. Powell · D. R. Liptzin (✉)
Department of Pediatrics, University of Washington, Seattle, WA, USA
e-mail: Weston.powell@seattlechildrens.org; Deborah.Liptzin@seattlechildrens.org

E. R. Swenson, A. M. Luks (eds.), *The Lungs at the Extremes of Environment and Age*, Respiratory Medicine, https://doi.org/10.1007/978-3-031-98371-9_7

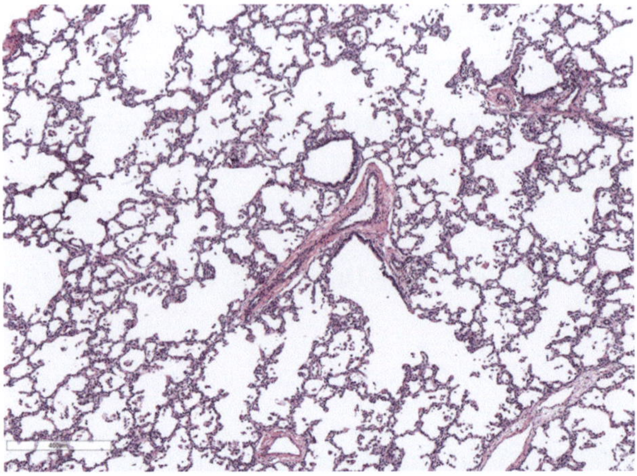

Fig. 7.1 Normal lung at term

tachypnea of the newborn (TTN), persistent pulmonary hypertension of the newborn (PPHN), bronchopulmonary dysplasia (BPD), and defects of lung development including congenital diaphragmatic hernia (CDH). We focus on the key areas of mechanics, pulmonary blood flow, and respiratory control to highlight the physiologic changes that occur in the neonate.

The First Breath

The first breath ex utero marks a fundamental and rapid shift in the physiology of the human lung. As eloquently described over 60 years ago:

> The infant is called on, in one sudden moment, to replace the gestational system of oxygen supply and carbon dioxide disposal by the placental circulation with a new system employing the hitherto unused lungs. How impressive this performance is cannot be appreciated until one examines the obstacles the baby must surmount in drawing its first breath. It is born with its lungs and air passages…distended by fluid, and against this and other resistances it must inflate the lungs, keep them inflated between breaths and quickly establish a breathing rhythm… Never again will it be obliged to draw air into a closed and resisting space [1].

Just prior to the moment of parturition, the fetal lungs are full of amniotic fluid; in fact, the volume of fetal lung fluid is greater than the functional residual capacity (FRC) established shortly after delivery [2, 3]. During the second half of gestation, the lung actively secretes fluid through epithelial chloride channels, and there is minimal reabsorption through epithelial sodium channels [3, 4]. Amniotic fluid distends the lungs and stimulates fetal lung development [3]. In addition to being fluid-filled, the fetal lungs experience respiratory movements that are vital to lung development; more of these movements occur in female than male fetuses [5, 6].

The fetal lung fluid must be cleared for postnatal gas exchange to occur. This occurs in the first 1–2 min of life across 40–50 respiratory cycles as demonstrated via electrical impedance tomography [7]. Historically, "vaginal squeeze" was thought to aid clearance of lung fluid (this was visualized by Warnekros via radiographs during birth in 1917), but this concept has fallen out of favor, especially as most infants delivered via cesarean section rather than vaginal delivery experience an uneventful transition [3, 8]. Fluid clearance occurs because the lung transitions from a secretory organ to an absorptive organ around the onset of labor [9]. Endogenous catecholamines and cortisol stop secretion of chloride into the alveoli shortly before delivery and upregulate the amiloride-sensitive apical epithelial sodium channels (ENaC) and basolateral sodium/potassium ATPase pump activity [3]. Sodium reabsorption at the apical surface of epithelial cells through ENaC is paired with basolateral secretion of sodium via a sodium/potassium ATPase, which establishes an electrochemical gradient across the epithelium with passive movement of chloride ions into the interstitium and an osmotic gradient to reabsorb fluid [4, 10, 11]. Glucocorticoids and vasopressin also stimulate transcription of ENaC [3]. Gene expression of ENaC increases during late gestation to facilitate transition to the ex utero environment.

In addition to the cellular mechanisms that drive alveolar fluid clearance, respiratory efforts of the newborn also aid in the transition to air-filled lungs. These efforts lead to rapid establishment of the aerated FRC; within the first five breaths, almost half of maximal FRC is achieved [7]. Recruiting aerated lung within those first few breaths occurs due to periods of crying associated with increased peak inspiratory flow during a short inhalation period followed by prolonged exhalation period (called "expiratory braking"). Often associated with grunting or crying, this leads to redistribution of air to nonrecruited regions and from centrally to distally within the lung [3, 7]. Expiratory braking is similar to what is seen in older infants who employ a similar mechanism to maintain FRC through an active process to slow exhalation. Fluid is also cleared from the lung interstitium, which creates more typical transalveolar pressures that help maintain the air-filled spaces. Measurement of interstitial pressure in animal models at birth demonstrates an increase in interstitial pressure soon after birth due to the rapid influx of more than 15 mL/kg of fluid. Over 4–6 h, the pressure becomes negative as the fluid drains through lymphatics [12]. The large negative inspiratory pressure (−40 to −60 cmH_2O) measured in infants after birth is necessary to overcome the poor compliance of the fluid-filled lung and facilitate ongoing clearance of pulmonary and interstitial fluid [13].

Mechanical Disadvantages in Infant Respiratory Mechanics

Infants require an extraordinary effort to establish FRC by about 1 min after parturition: Using esophageal probes, the first breath requires up to −60 cmH_2O to achieve a 40 mL breath [1, 7, 14].

Postnatally, the infant respiratory system is at a mechanical disadvantage. While a highly compliant chest wall eases passage through the birth canal [15], it contributes to FRC being barely above residual volume. A lower FRC results as chest wall recoil is reduced in the setting of a more compliant chest wall, while lung compliance remains normal to decreased in the early neonatal period from pulmonary fluid. Additional perturbations to the system (e.g., bronchiolitis, aspiration, and delayed transition) can lead to greater risk for atelectasis. Infants primarily increase minute ventilation by increasing the respiratory rate with smaller changes in tidal volume; in older children and adults, minute ventilation is increased primarily by increasing tidal volume and the respiratory rate.

Infants use active glottic narrowing to slow exhalation (called laryngeal braking or expiratory braking) to increase intrapulmonary pressures and, therefore, maintain FRC for up to the first year, similar to respiratory patterns seen at birth as discussed above [3, 7, 16]. Crying and grunting are one form of expiratory braking: The first cry likely serves to establish FRC; preterm infants use more expiratory braking than their full-term counterparts to maintain FRC [3]. Chest wall compliance becomes equal to lung compliance at around age 2 [15].

The conformation of the ribcage itself also influences how infants breathe. As Smith reported, "the baby's chest has a shape rather more like that of a cone than that of a cylinder, with its ribs lowered like the ribs of an incompletely opened umbrella. As the breathing movement begins the chest narrows slightly in transverse diameter…at the end point of expiration the lungs still contain a large amount of air" [1]. Infant ribs are positioned more horizontally, so the zone of apposition of the diaphragm is smaller, leading to a mechanical disadvantage for inhalation [17]. In infants, the rib cage contributes only one-third of tidal volume changes during breathing, and increases to two-thirds in older children [17, 18]. The adult—or more mechanically efficient—configuration with ribs at an oblique angle is achieved by age 2 [19] due to postnatal effects of gravity, improved muscle tone (especially intercostals and abdominals), and bone mineralization [17].

There are additional proximal structural differences in infants compared to older children and adults. Infants breathe preferentially through the nose to best coordinate feeding and breathing [20]. The larynx is more proximal in infants than older children and adults. This helps make a seal for feeding but can also lead to more upper airway obstruction. Around age 2, there is a major conformational change to better allow for speech [16].

In summary, adequately recruiting and aerating the lung is critical for the transition to postnatal physiology as fluid-filled lungs have lower compliance and higher airway resistance compared to aerated lungs. Multiple processes, including epithelial fluid transport, airway recruitment through the first few breaths of life, and clearance of interstitial fluid, are best understood as a multiple-phase process that occurs in a nonhomogeneous manner across the lung [21].

Pulmonary Circulation Transition

Coinciding with the first breaths, the pulmonary vasculature also undergoes an extraordinary transition. In the fetal circulation, pulmonary vascular resistance (PVR) and pressures are high to limit blood from perfusing the unventilated and growing lungs, which may not be ready to handle the entire cardiac output. The high PVR, combined with right-to-left shunting through the foramen ovale and ductus arteriosus, and low systemic vascular resistance permit high blood flow to the placenta for gas exchange, nutrient uptake, and waste removal. These high pulmonary pressures result from increased vascular tone mediated by vasoconstrictors such as endothelin and thromboxane as well as local hypercapnia and physical compression of pulmonary capillaries by the fluid-filled lung [22, 23]. In the instant of parturition, the pulmonary vascular resistance decreases nearly fivefold (from 0.4 mmHg/mL\L/min/kg to 0.08 mmHg/mL/min/kg), thereby allowing increased pulmonary blood flow and initiation of pulmonary gas exchange [22, 24]. The drop in pulmonary vascular resistance occurs due to a combination of changes in mechanical forces on the vascular bed and vasodilatory remodeling. As lung aeration occurs, pulmonary vascular pressure falls and the lung is stretched to FRC, thus leading to release of mechanical compression of the vascular bed by a fluid-filled lung. Simultaneously, the increase in oxygen tension leads to release of vasodilators, such as endothelium-derived nitric oxide, prostacyclin, cyclic guanosine monophosphate, and cyclic adenosine monophosphate [22, 23]. Hypoxic pulmonary vasoconstriction or oxygen-dependent vasodilation appears only very late in gestation and does not contribute to the high PVR [25]. As a result, the lungs become a low-resistance circuit to accept the entire cardiac output and assume the role of gas exchange from the placenta.

When Things Go Wrong

Many factors need to line up for a fetus to survive to parturition with functioning lungs. First, a fertilized egg must implant and progress through the early embryologic stages of development. The lungs must then progress through the canalicular, saccular, pseudoglandular, and alveolar stages of development to prepare for delivery at term with successful transition to the extrauterine environment. Even when a fetus survives the early embryologic stages and the remainder of pregnancy, many intrauterine or extrauterine factors can prevent a normal transition. The various conditions that result from difficulty transitioning to postnatal life highlight the complex and dynamic physiologic changes that occur during early postnatal life.

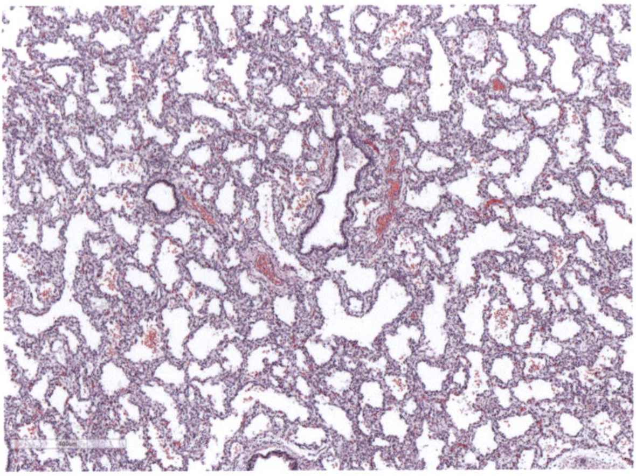

Fig. 7.2 Pulmonary hyperplasia in a second trimester fetus with laryngeal atresia/CHAOS characterized by a marked increase in the number of immature alveolar spaces

When Things Go Wrong: Fluid

Too Much Lung Fluid In Utero

If the upper airway is occluded such as in congenital high airway obstruction syndrome (CHAOS), secreted fluid is trapped in the lungs, leading to dysfunction in other organs, such as heart failure and/or fetal hydrops [26]. The lungs are typically about twice the normal weight and are more developed than expected for gestational age (Fig. 7.2) [27]. Complete airway obstruction is not survivable, but ex utero intrapartum tracheostomy can sustain life [28]. Similarly, congenital lymphatic malformations, polyhydramnios due to congenital anomalies, neonatal heart failure, maternal diabetes, alloimmunization, infection, or idiopathic causes may lead to excess body and lung fluid at birth, which impairs the transition to an air-filled lung [29].

Too Little Lung Fluid In Utero

Lung development is also compromised by insufficient amniotic fluid production [30, 31]. Potter's syndrome, or bilateral renal agenesis, results in inadequate urine production and severe oligohydramnios, and subsequently in utero thoracic compression, reduced fetal breathing volumes, and pulmonary hypoplasia that is incompatible with extrauterine life (Fig. 7.3) [30]. In congenital diaphragmatic hernia (CDH), lung development is impaired, primarily on the ipsilateral side to the hernia (Fig. 7.4), but also on the contralateral side [31–34]. Based on evidence from animal models showing lung overgrowth following tracheal ligation, attempts have been made to palliate CDH-related pulmonary hypoplasia with temporary tracheal

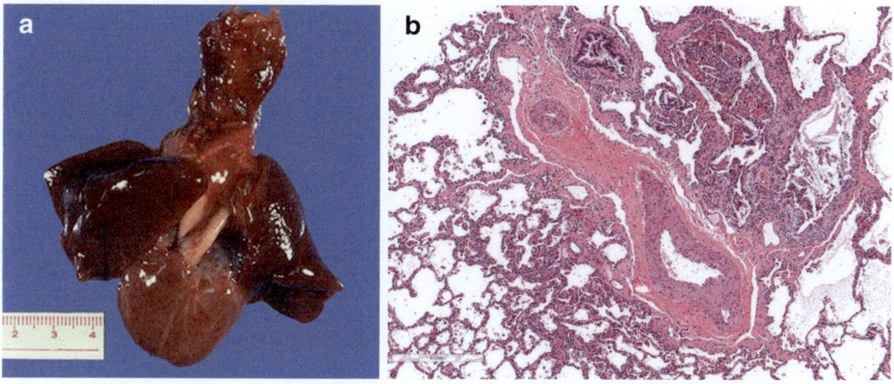

Fig. 7.3 (**a**) Gross pathology findings of severe pulmonary hypoplasia in bladder outlet obstruction. (**b**) Histologic correlate of pulmonary hypoplasia in the setting of oligohydramnios with enlarged alveolar spaces lacking secondary septa, interstitial fibrosis, and dramatic pulmonary vascular remodeling reflective of pulmonary arterial hypertension

Fig. 7.4 Congenital diaphragmatic hernia with gross pulmonary hypoplasia on the ipsilateral side to the hernia (right side of image)

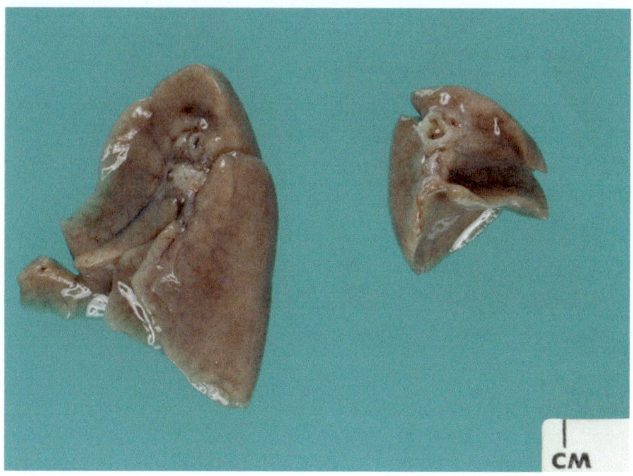

occlusion, but long-term results have been disappointing except in a limited number of cases [35–39]. Pulmonary hypoplasia can also develop due to thoracic dystrophy [40].

Too Much Fluid in the Lungs Postpartum

Much more commonly, the postpartum transition is impaired due to delayed clearance of fetal lung fluid, leading to tachypnea within the first 6 h of delivery, a problem referred to as transient tachypnea of the newborn (TTN). Newborns with TTN breathe 80–140 breaths per minute with or without grunting within the first 6 h of life. Chest radiographs demonstrate a large cardiac silhouette and prominent markings branching out from hila suggestive of vascular engorgement [41]. Treatment is supportive, including respiratory support and avoidance of oral feeding. TTN resolves within the first few days of life. In placebo-controlled trials, neither furosemide nor epinephrine hastens recovery [42, 43].

When Things Go Wrong: Prematurity

Beyond oligohydramnios and thoracic compression, the more common cause of lung hypoplasia is prematurity, or bronchopulmonary dysplasia (BPD). Infants born early can suffer from lung hypoplasia, vascular immaturity, and surfactant deficiency (Fig. 7.5) with increasing difficulty the earlier an infant is born.

In 1967, Northway described bronchopulmonary dysplasia, a chronic pulmonary disease following oxygen toxicity for treatment of hyaline membrane disease (also known as respiratory distress syndrome (RDS) or surfactant deficiency) [44]. Surfactant, primarily composed of phospholipid (dipalmitoylphosphatidylcholine), decreases the surface tension of alveoli, preventing alveolar atelectasis [45]. Type II alveolar epithelial cells start producing surfactant at 5–7 months' gestation [45, 46]. Respiratory distress syndrome or hyaline membrane disease is demonstrated in Fig. 7.6 with the eponymous hyaline membranes. Risk factors for development of BPD include prematurity, inflammation (such as from chorioamnionitis), oxygen toxicity, sepsis, and/or positive pressure ventilation [46]. BPD is currently defined as requiring respiratory support at 36 weeks' postmenstrual age [47]. This definition was developed from a cohort of children born at less than 27 weeks' gestation and was based on the measures that best predicted death after 36 weeks' postmenstrual age or adverse respiratory and neurodevelopmental outcomes in toddlerhood [47].

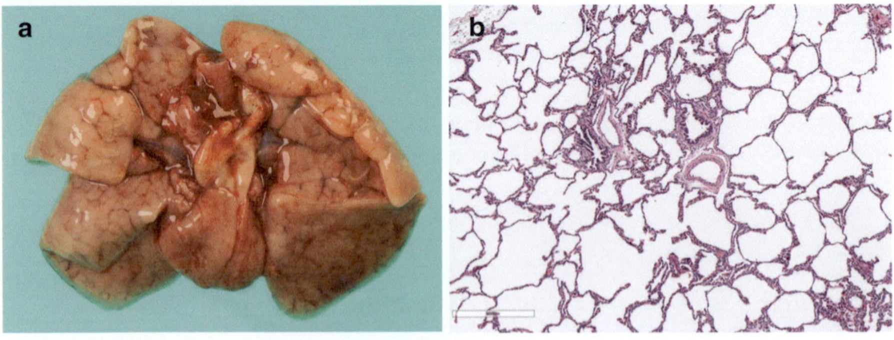

Fig. 7.5 (**a**) Gross findings of bronchopulmonary dysplasia and diffuse lobar hyperinflation in an infant born at 23 weeks' gestation after treatment with chronic ventilation. (**b**) Histologic correlate of bronchopulmonary dysplasia with markedly enlarged simplified alveolar spaces resulting in reduced surface area for gas exchange

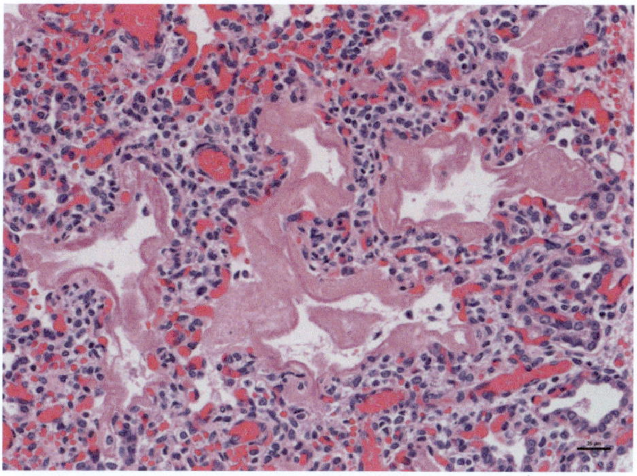

Fig. 7.6 Respiratory distress syndrome in a 30-week gestation neonate after a pregnancy complicated by oligohydramnios. Classic findings of severely congested and immature alveolar spaces lined by eosinophilic hyaline membranes are demonstrated

Of 351 infants born prior to 32 weeks' gestation and hospitalized across eight neonatal intensive care units in the United States, 36.5% met criteria for severe BPD [48]. Of infants born in Norway at less than 30 weeks' gestation, 67.3% developed BPD [49].

Glucocorticoids accelerate lung development including surfactant production and can be given prenatally or postnatally [46]. Exogenous surfactant allows premature neonates to survive RDS [46]. Ventilation strategies including avoidance of hyperoxia and intubation have decreased the risk of BPD [46].

When Things Go Wrong: Surfactant Dysfunction

Pulmonary surfactant is primarily composed of phospholipids (which comprise exogenous surfactant), but 10–20% of surfactant is comprised of proteins. In addition to phospholipids, endogenous pulmonary surfactant also contains proteins that are essential to surfactant processing, function, and degradation. A number of mutations in surfactant protein production and metabolism lead to pulmonary alveolar proteinosis, widened interstitium, and type II alveolar epithelial cell hyperplasia, and, as a result, poor lung compliance and respiratory failure [50]. Neonates with *ABCA3* Null/Null mutations and *SFTPB* mutations present with severe respiratory failure in the neonatal period, for which lung transplantation is the only suitable intervention [51, 52] (Fig. 7.7). Other mutations in surfactant production and metabolism, such as *ABCA3*, *NKX2*-1, *SFTPC*, and *GM-CSF*-associated mutations, can present later in infancy and even in adolescence or adulthood with variable histologic findings [52].

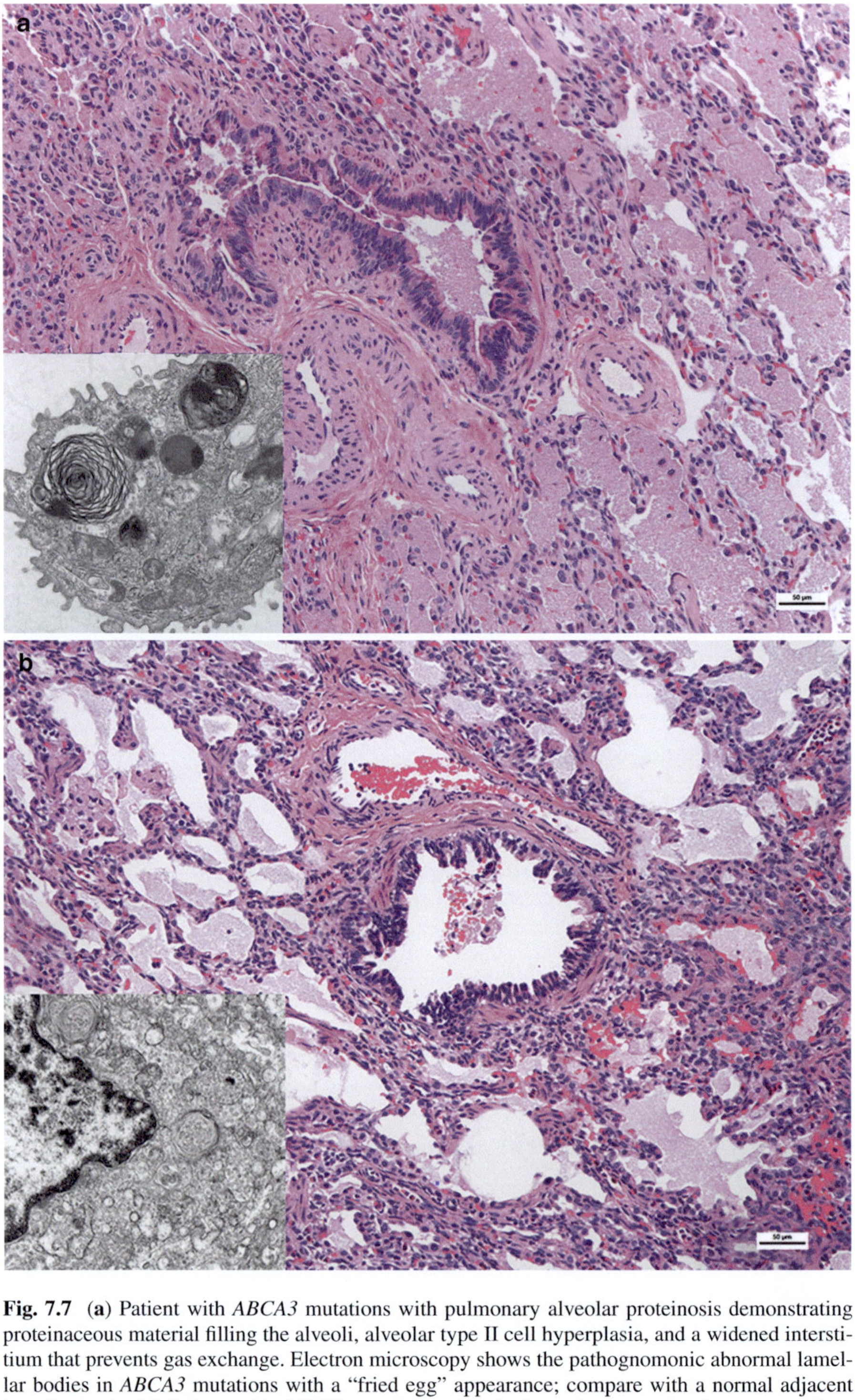

Fig. 7.7 (**a**) Patient with *ABCA3* mutations with pulmonary alveolar proteinosis demonstrating proteinaceous material filling the alveoli, alveolar type II cell hyperplasia, and a widened interstitium that prevents gas exchange. Electron microscopy shows the pathognomonic abnormal lamellar bodies in *ABCA3* mutations with a "fried egg" appearance; compare with a normal adjacent lamellar body. (**b**) Patient with *SFTPB* mutations with similar pulmonary alveolar proteinosis to (**a**) but complete absence of normal lamellar bodies on electron microscopy

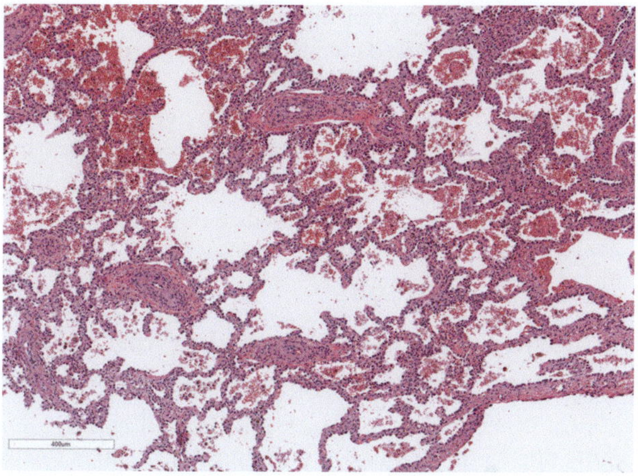

Fig. 7.8 Patient with Trisomy 21 with severe pulmonary arterial vascular remodeling accompanying deficient alveolar growth

When Things Go Wrong: Pulmonary Hypertension

When pulmonary vascular pressures do not fall appropriately, neonates develop respiratory distress and hypoxemia, a problem known as persistent pulmonary hypertension of the newborn (PPHN) [23]. Risk factors for PPHN include maternal diabetes, meconium aspiration, and oligohydramnios/pulmonary hypoplasia, although many cases are idiopathic [23]. Figures 7.3a and 7.8 demonstrate severe pulmonary arterial vascular remodeling consistent with pulmonary hypertension. Treatment includes cardiorespiratory support such as oxygen, ventilation, and extracorporeal membrane oxygenation, as well as pharmacologic pulmonary vasodilators [23, 53].

When Things Go Wrong: Airway Edema

Bronchiolitis is a leading cause of respiratory morbidity and mortality in young children [54]. While respiratory syncytial virus is the primary cause, any respiratory virus can trigger distal bronchiolar inflammation [54]. Young children are particularly susceptible to severe disease due to the small diameter of infant bronchioles. Given that airway resistance is inversely related to the radius to the fourth power, even a slight decrease in bronchiolar radius—due to, for example, airway mucosal edema—leads to a significantly greater increase in airway resistance than in adults [55]. The highly compliant chest wall and suboptimal respiratory mechanics further contribute to respiratory distress in such cases.

Croup or acute laryngotracheitis presents in young children, more commonly in males than females [56]. The classic presentation is a toddler who goes to bed either completely healthy or with a slight runny nose, and then awakens in the middle of the night with a barky cough and terrifying stridor [57]. Again, given that airway resistance is inversely related to the radius to the fourth power, even a slight decrease in laryngeal radius leads to a significantly greater increase in airway resistance than in adults [55]. As such narrowing occurs in the larger airways where turbulent flow occurs, the driving pressure required to overcome the increase in resistance increases exponentially, leading to the markedly increased work of breathing seen in children. As younger children have impaired mechanics (as discussed above), they are at risk for rapid decompensation if they tire out.

Immature Control of Breathing and Sleep

Control of breathing in infants during wakefulness and sleep differs from that of adults due to differences in both lung mechanics (as discussed above) and chemosensitivity. As a result, infants are more prone to breathing instability with altered loop gain leading to episodes of periodic breathing. Periodic breathing (at least two pauses of 3–6 s within a 20-s epoch) occurs more frequently in infancy [58]. Such instability occurs primarily early in the postnatal period as 78% of newborns experience periodic breathing in the first 2 weeks of life, while only 29% of infants demonstrated periodic breathing at 39–52 weeks [59]. Periodic breathing is thought to be secondary to altered chemoreceptor sensitivity, leading to overcompensation for changes in partial pressures of CO_2, and resulting in alternating periods of tachypnea and apnea [59, 60].

The altered chemosensitivity is likely due to immaturity of both central and peripheral chemoreceptors, leading to labile ventilatory responses to CO_2 and O_2 [61]. In animals, the response to CO_2 is reduced within the first few days of life as compared to 2 weeks later [62]. Similarly, premature infants have decreased central chemosensitivity to CO_2 over the first 5 weeks of life [63]. Such decreased chemosensitivity partially explains the apnea seen in premature infants which usually resolves by corrected gestational age of 40–44 weeks as ventilation increases more slowly with rising CO_2. The ventilatory response to O_2 is low immediately after birth and then rapidly rises over the first few weeks of life coinciding with observed cellular changes in the carotid body [61, 64]. Infants demonstrate a biphasic ventilatory response to hypoxemia with an immediate 60–120-s increase in ventilation followed by a subsequent decrease in ventilation and occasionally subsequent apneas [16]. Conversely, a period of hyperoxia leads to decreased ventilation initially followed by a subsequent increase in ventilation and risk for apneas [65]. At higher elevation (3100 m), the response may be more complex with an initial decrease in ventilation, followed by a subsequent increase and then a progressive decrease [66].

In adults, the combined impact of O_2 and CO_2 on ventilatory responses leads to an integrated response with a “multiplicative” controller, such that the response to hypoxemia and hypercapnia is greater than the sum of either individual response and allows for a stable apneic threshold as the slope of the ventilatory response curve changes with hypoxia or hyperoxia. In contrast, an additive controller leads to rightward or leftward shift of the ventilatory response to hypoxemia or hyperoxia, but not a change in slope resulting in a labile apneic threshold [61]. The additive response helps explain why hyperoxia can induce apneic events in infants as the ventilatory drive from O_2 is eliminated and the CO_2 response is diminished [65]. Babies born prematurely experience more apnea: Caffeine, an adenosine antagonist, combats apnea of prematurity by stimulating the medulla's respiratory center and subsequently increasing diaphragmatic activity and tidal volume [67, 68] Caffeine has also been shown to decrease rates of bronchopulmonary dysplasia [69].

Alteration in control of breathing during infancy is often used to explain clinical syndromes involving apnea found during the first year of life. Two such syndromes are "Brief, Resolved, Unexplained Events" termed BRUEs (formerly called "Apparent Life-Threatening Events"—ALTEs) and "Sudden Unexplained Infant Death Syndrome" (SUIDS or SIDS). BRUEs are characterized by (1) cyanosis or pallor; (2) absent, decreased, or irregular breathing; (3) marked change in tone; and (4) altered level of responsiveness as a sudden, brief, and resolved episode in infants less than 1 year of age [70]. While BRUEs are defined by the absence of other clear explanation or diagnosis, the propensity of infants to have more unstable breathing in response to smaller stimuli could provide one explanation for why BRUEs are restricted to those less than 1 year of age. In 2016, the American Academy of Pediatrics proposed BRUE as an alternative to provide a clearer definition rather than the broader, ill-defined ALTE. The development of a definition for ALTE originated in the 1980s to distinguish such events as distinct and separate from SUIDS [71]. As diagnosis of SUIDS requires the absence of a clear pathogenic or histopathological explanation postmortem, establishing a clear pathophysiology is not possible. Given the historical connection among these three definitions, the "unexplained" conventional histopathology has led to proposed hypotheses reliant on the differences in reflexes and ventilatory control found during the first year of life. Such differences during the first year of life are thought to contribute to a "triple-risk" model for SUIDS by providing a rational basis for the period of greatest vulnerability (greatest in the first few months of life and decreasing risk over the first year of life) [72]. Ultimately, while understanding breathing control during infancy provides some insight into SUIDS, the underlying causes of SUIDS are likely multifactorial, including individual genetic/metabolic risk factors in infancy, exogenous and environmental factors, and the critical period of vulnerability during the first year of life.

Challenges arise in integrating the behavioral and breathing interventions in sleep-related breathing disorders as developmental considerations differ across childhood. In children, an obstructive apnea–hypopnea index of one or greater is consistent with obstructive sleep apnea (OSA), whereas in adults, the cutoff is five events per hour [73]. Some studies suggest using an obstructive apnea–hypopnea index of two or greater [74]. Children must have snoring, labored/obstructed breathing, and/or daytime consequences such as sleepiness or hyperactivity [73]. Anatomically, children have increased upper airway space competition: Upper airway lymphoid tissue increases during the first decade, but bony structures are slower to grow, causing the tonsils and adenoids to occupy proportionally more space in the proximal airway [16].

In children, males and females are equally likely to suffer from adenotonsillar hypertrophy, and symptoms from obstructive sleep apnea can include anything on the weight spectrum from failure to thrive to obesity [16]. Children with obstructive sleep apnea typically have less daytime sleepiness than adults but demonstrate hyperactivity and/or developmental delay [16]. While continuous positive airway pressure (CPAP) is a cornerstone for treatment of OSA in adults, finding a suitable mask interface is much more challenging in children due to the spectrum of head and face structures that an individual has from infancy to postpuberty. Similarly, behavioral difficulties make adherence to CPAP much more challenging. Furthermore, as craniofacial structures are still developing throughout childhood, chronic therapy with CPAP in young children may carry the added risk of midface remodeling. Medications, such as intranasal steroids and montelukast, and adenotonsillectomy are typically first-line approaches to OSA in children [75]. When surgical intervention (tonsillectomy and adenoidectomy) was compared to watchful waiting, children who underwent earlier surgical intervention had improved behavior, quality of life, and symptom reduction [74].

Conclusion

The transition from intrauterine to extrauterine life is a dramatic process rife with opportunities for problems. Fortunately, in the majority of infants, such transition proceeds uneventfully, but the consequences of altered mechanics, blood flow, and respiratory control help explain many observations seen in respiratory function in healthy infants. The observed differences in physiology in the neonatal and infant lung as compared to the adult pulmonary system highlight why infants are at increased risk for certain complications and disease states. Small differences in the smaller airways of children lead to exponentially larger problems. Understanding the evolving physiology throughout the neonatal period is critical for pediatricians and others caring for these infants.

References

1. Smith CA. The first breath. Sci Am. 1963;209:27–35.
2. Harding R, Hooper SB. Regulation of lung expansion and lung growth before birth. J Appl Physiol (1985). 1996;81(1):209–24.
3. te Pas AB, Wong C, Kamlin CO, Dawson JA, Morley CJ, Davis PG. Breathing patterns in preterm and term infants immediately after birth. Pediatr Res. 2009;65(3):352–6.
4. Matalon S, Bartoszewski R, Collawn JF. Role of epithelial sodium channels in the regulation of lung fluid homeostasis. Am J Physiol Lung Cell Mol Physiol. 2015;309(11):L1229–38.

5. Harding R. Fetal pulmonary development: the role of respiratory movements. Equine Vet J Suppl. 1997;24:32–9.
6. Hepper PG, Shannon EA, Dornan JC. Sex differences in fetal mouth movements. Lancet. 1997;350(9094):1820.
7. Tingay DG, Farrell O, Thomson J, Perkins EJ, Pereira-Fantini PM, Waldmann AD, et al. Imaging the respiratory transition at birth: unraveling the complexities of the first breaths of life. Am J Respir Crit Care Med. 2021;204(1):82–91.
8. Bland RD. Loss of liquid from the lung lumen in labor: more than a simple "squeeze". Am J Physiol Lung Cell Mol Physiol. 2001;280(4):L602–5.
9. Lines A, Hooper SB, Harding R. Lung liquid production rates and volumes do not decrease before labor in healthy fetal sheep. J Appl Physiol (1985). 1997;82(3):927–32.
10. Jain L, Eaton DC. Alveolar fluid transport: a changing paradigm. Am J Physiol Lung Cell Mol Physiol. 2006;290(4):L646–8.
11. Siew ML, Wallace MJ, Kitchen MJ, Lewis RA, Fouras A, Te Pas AB, et al. Inspiration regulates the rate and temporal pattern of lung liquid clearance and lung aeration at birth. J Appl Physiol (1985). 2009;106(6):1888–95.
12. Miserocchi G, Poskurica BH, Del Fabbro M. Pulmonary interstitial pressure in anesthetized paralyzed newborn rabbits. J Appl Physiol (1985). 1994;77(5):2260–8.
13. Vyas H, Milner AD, Hopkins IE. Intrathoracic pressure and volume changes during the spontaneous onset of respiration in babies born by cesarean section and by vaginal delivery. J Pediatr. 1981;99(5):787–91.
14. Milner AD, Sauders RA. Pressure and volume changes during the first breath of human neonates. Arch Dis Child. 1977;52(12):918–24.
15. Papastamelos C, Panitch HB, England SE, Allen JL. Developmental changes in chest wall compliance in infancy and early childhood. J Appl Physiol (1985). 1995;78(1):179–84.
16. Marcus CL. Sleep-disordered breathing in children. Am J Respir Crit Care Med. 2001;164(1):16–30.
17. Hershenson MB, Colin AA, Wohl ME, Stark AR. Changes in the contribution of the rib cage to tidal breathing during infancy. Am Rev Respir Dis. 1990;141(4 Pt 1):922–5.
18. Tabachnik E, Muller NL, Bryan AC, Levison H. Changes in ventilation and chest wall mechanics during sleep in normal adolescents. J Appl Physiol Respir Environ Exerc Physiol. 1981;51(3):557–64.
19. Openshaw P, Edwards S, Helms P. Changes in rib cage geometry during childhood. Thorax. 1984;39(8):624–7.
20. Miller MJ, Martin RJ, Carlo WA, Fouke JM, Strohl KP, Fanaroff AA. Oral breathing in newborn infants. J Pediatr. 1985;107(3):465–9.
21. Hooper SB, Te Pas AB, Kitchen MJ. Respiratory transition in the newborn: a three-phase process. Arch Dis Child Fetal Neonatal Ed. 2016;101(3):F266–71.
22. Gao Y, Raj JU. Regulation of the pulmonary circulation in the fetus and newborn. Physiol Rev. 2010;90(4):1291–335.
23. Mandell E, Kinsella JP, Abman SH. Persistent pulmonary hypertension of the newborn. Pediatr Pulmonol. 2021;56(3):661–9.
24. Heymann MA. Control of the pulmonary circulation in the fetus and during the transitional period to air breathing. Eur J Obstet Gynecol Reprod Biol. 1999;84(2):127–32.
25. Morin FC, Egan EA. Pulmonary hemodynamics in fetal lambs during development at normal and increased oxygen tension. J Appl Physiol (1985). 1992;73(1):213–8.
26. Hedrick MH, Ferro MM, Filly RA, Flake AW, Harrison MR, Adzick NS. Congenital high airway obstruction syndrome (CHAOS): a potential for perinatal intervention. J Pediatr Surg. 1994;29(2):271–4.
27. Wigglesworth JS, Desai R, Hislop AA. Fetal lung growth in congenital laryngeal atresia. Pediatr Pathol. 1987;7(5–6):515–25.

28. DeCou JM, Jones DC, Jacobs HD, Touloukian RJ. Successful ex utero intrapartum treatment (EXIT) procedure for congenital high airway obstruction syndrome (CHAOS) owing to laryngeal atresia. J Pediatr Surg. 1998;33(10):1563–5.
29. Pagan M, Magann EF, Rabie N, Steelman SC, Hu Z, Ounpraseuth S. Idiopathic polyhydramnios and pregnancy outcome: systematic review and meta-analysis. Ultrasound Obstet Gynecol. 2023;61(3):302–9.
30. Thomas IT, Smith DW. Oligohydramnios, cause of the nonrenal features of Potter's syndrome, including pulmonary hypoplasia. J Pediatr. 1974;84(6):811–5.
31. Ameis D, Khoshgoo N, Keijzer R. Abnormal lung development in congenital diaphragmatic hernia. Semin Pediatr Surg. 2017;26(3):123–8.
32. Moya FR, Thomas VL, Romaguera J, Mysore MR, Maberry M, Bernard A, et al. Fetal lung maturation in congenital diaphragmatic hernia. Am J Obstet Gynecol. 1995;173(5):1401–5.
33. Beals DA, Schloo BL, Vacanti JP, Reid LM, Wilson JM. Pulmonary growth and remodeling in infants with high-risk congenital diaphragmatic hernia. J Pediatr Surg. 1992;27(8):997–1001; discussion −2.
34. Chinoy MR. Pulmonary hypoplasia and congenital diaphragmatic hernia: advances in the pathogenetics and regulation of lung development. J Surg Res. 2002;106(1):209–23.
35. Hedrick MH, Estes JM, Sullivan KM, Bealer JF, Kitterman JA, Flake AW, et al. Plug the lung until it grows (PLUG): a new method to treat congenital diaphragmatic hernia in utero. J Pediatr Surg. 1994;29(5):612–7.
36. Flake AW, Crombleholme TM, Johnson MP, Howell LJ, Adzick NS. Treatment of severe congenital diaphragmatic hernia by fetal tracheal occlusion: clinical experience with fifteen cases. Am J Obstet Gynecol. 2000;183(5):1059–66.
37. Skarsgard ED, Meuli M, VanderWall KJ, Bealer JF, Adzick NS, Harrison MR. Fetal endoscopic tracheal occlusion ('Fetendo-PLUG') for congenital diaphragmatic hernia. J Pediatr Surg. 1996;31(10):1335–8.
38. Bohn D. Congenital diaphragmatic hernia. Am J Respir Crit Care Med. 2002;166(7):911–5.
39. Chatterjee D, Ing RJ, Gien J. Update on congenital diaphragmatic hernia. Anesth Analg. 2020;131(3):808–21.
40. Inselman LS, Mellins RB. Growth and development of the lung. J Pediatr. 1981;98(1):1–15.
41. Avery ME, Gatewood OB, Brumley G. Transient tachypnea of newborn. Possible delayed resorption of fluid at birth. Am J Dis Child. 1966;111(4):380–5.
42. Kao B, Stewart de Ramirez SA, Belfort MB, Hansen A. Inhaled epinephrine for the treatment of transient tachypnea of the newborn. J Perinatol. 2008;28(3):205–10.
43. Wiswell TE, Rawlings JS, Smith FR, Goo ED. Effect of furosemide on the clinical course of transient tachypnea of the newborn. Pediatrics. 1985;75(5):908–10.
44. Northway WH, Rosan RC, Porter DY. Pulmonary disease following respirator therapy of hyaline-membrane disease. Bronchopulmonary dysplasia. N Engl J Med. 1967;276(7):357–68.
45. Clements JA. Surface tension in the lungs. Sci Am. 1962;207:120–30.
46. Thébaud B, Goss KN, Laughon M, Whitsett JA, Abman SH, Steinhorn RH, et al. Bronchopulmonary dysplasia. Nat Rev Dis Primers. 2019;5(1):78.
47. Jensen EA, Dysart K, Gantz MG, McDonald S, Bamat NA, Keszler M, et al. The diagnosis of bronchopulmonary dysplasia in very preterm infants. An evidence-based approach. Am J Respir Crit Care Med. 2019;200(6):751–9.
48. Guaman MC, Gien J, Baker CD, Zhang H, Austin ED, Collaco JM. Point prevalence, clinical characteristics, and treatment variation for infants with severe bronchopulmonary dysplasia. Am J Perinatol. 2015;32(10):960–7.
49. Farstad T, Bratlid D, Medbo S, Markestad T. Bronchopulmonary dysplasia—prevalence, severity and predictive factors in a national cohort of extremely premature infants. Acta Paediatr. 2011;100(1):53–8.
50. Nogee LM. Genetic causes of surfactant protein abnormalities. Curr Opin Pediatr. 2019;31(3):330–9.

51. Wambach JA, Casey AM, Fishman MP, Wegner DJ, Wert SE, Cole FS, et al. Genotype-phenotype correlations for infants and children with ABCA3 deficiency. Am J Respir Crit Care Med. 2014;189(12):1538–43.
52. Wert SE, Whitsett JA, Nogee LM. Genetic disorders of surfactant dysfunction. Pediatr Dev Pathol. 2009;12(4):253–74.
53. Kinsella JP, Neish SR, Ivy DD, Shaffer E, Abman SH. Clinical responses to prolonged treatment of persistent pulmonary hypertension of the newborn with low doses of inhaled nitric oxide. J Pediatr. 1993;123(1):103–8.
54. Dalziel SR, Haskell L, O'Brien S, Borland ML, Plint AC, Babl FE, et al. Bronchiolitis. Lancet. 2022;400(10349):392–406.
55. Wohl ME, Chernick V. State of the art: bronchiolitis. Am Rev Respir Dis. 1978;118(4):759–81.
56. Liptzin DR, Landau LI, Taussig LM. Sex and the lung: observations, hypotheses, and future directions. Pediatr Pulmonol. 2015;50(12):1159–69.
57. Cherry JD. Clinical practice. Croup. N Engl J Med. 2008;358(4):384–91.
58. Hoppenbrouwers T, Hodgman JE, Harper RM, Hofmann E, Sterman MB, McGinty DJ. Polygraphic studies of normal infants during the first six months of life: III. Incidence of apnea and periodic breathing. Pediatrics. 1977;60(4):418–25.
59. Kelly DH, Stellwagen LM, Kaitz E, Shannon DC. Apnea and periodic breathing in normal full-term infants during the first twelve months. Pediatr Pulmonol. 1985;1(4):215–9.
60. Patel M, Mohr M, Lake D, Delos J, Moorman JR, Sinkin RA, et al. Clinical associations with immature breathing in preterm infants: part 2-periodic breathing. Pediatr Res. 2016;80(1):28–34.
61. Edwards BA, Sands SA, Berger PJ. Postnatal maturation of breathing stability and loop gain: the role of carotid chemoreceptor development. Respir Physiol Neurobiol. 2013;185(1):144–55.
62. Bamford OS, Sterni LM, Wasicko MJ, Montrose MH, Carroll JL. Postnatal maturation of carotid body and type I cell chemoreception in the rat. Am J Phys. 1999;276(5):L875–84.
63. Rigatto H, Brady JP, de la Torre Verduzco R. Chemoreceptor reflexes in preterm infants: II. The effect of gestational and postnatal age on the ventilatory response to inhaled carbon dioxide. Pediatrics. 1975;55(5):614–20.
64. Søvik S, Lossius K, Eriksen M, Grøgaard J, Walløe L. Development of oxygen sensitivity in infants of smoking and non-smoking mothers. Early Hum Dev. 1999;56(2–3):217–32.
65. Haider AZ, Rehan V, Al-Saedi S, Alvaro R, Kwiatkowski K, Cates D, et al. Effect of baseline oxygenation on the ventilatory response to inhaled 100% oxygen in preterm infants. J Appl Physiol (1985). 1995;79(6):2101–5.
66. Cotton EK, Grunstein MM. Effects of hypoxia on respiratory control in neonates at high altitude. J Appl Physiol Respir Environ Exerc Physiol. 1980;48(4):587–95.
67. Kraaijenga JV, Hutten GJ, de Jongh FH, van Kaam AH. The effect of caffeine on diaphragmatic activity and tidal volume in preterm infants. J Pediatr. 2015;167(1):70–5.
68. Comer AM, Perry CM, Figgitt DP. Caffeine citrate: a review of its use in apnoea of prematurity. Paediatr Drugs. 2001;3(1):61–79.
69. Schmidt B, Roberts RS, Davis P, Doyle LW, Barrington KJ, Ohlsson A, et al. Caffeine therapy for apnea of prematurity. N Engl J Med. 2006;354(20):2112–21.
70. Tieder JS, Bonkowsky JL, Etzel RA, Franklin WH, Gremse DA, Herman B, et al. Brief resolved unexplained events (formerly apparent life-threatening events) and evaluation of lower-risk infants. Pediatrics. 2016;137(5)
71. National Institutes of Health Consensus Development Conference on Infantile Apnea and Home Monitoring, Sept 29 to Oct 1, 1986. Pediatrics. 1987;79(2):292–9.
72. Filiano JJ, Kinney HC. A perspective on neuropathologic findings in victims of the sudden infant death syndrome: the triple-risk model. Biol Neonate. 1994;65(3–4):194–7.
73. Medicine AAoS. International classification of sleep disorders. 3rd ed. Medicine AAoS, editor. Darien, IL; 2014.

74. Marcus CL, Moore RH, Rosen CL, Giordani B, Garetz SL, Taylor HG, et al. A randomized trial of adenotonsillectomy for childhood sleep apnea. N Engl J Med. 2013;368(25):2366–76.
75. Liming BJ, Ryan M, Mack D, Ahmad I, Camacho M. Montelukast and nasal corticosteroids to treat pediatric obstructive sleep apnea: a systematic review and meta-analysis. Otolaryngol Head Neck Surg. 2019;160(4):594–602.

Chapter 8
The Elderly Lung and Breathing

Harold L. Manning

This chapter focuses on changes in breathing that accompany aging. Several aspects of breathing will be considered, including the effects of aging on respiratory mechanics, respiratory muscle function, control of breathing, respiratory sensation, and pulmonary function tests.

Challenges in Studying Aging

There are several challenges in defining the effects of aging on breathing. First, many of the studies, particularly some of the earliest studies, included small numbers of subjects, with very few subjects at the true extremes of age. Thus, it is unclear in some studies whether failure to identify an effect of aging was due to a true absence of effect or simply an underpowered study with small numbers of subjects. Second, many of the studies included predominantly or even exclusively white male subjects, and the extent to which the findings can be generalized to the broader population is uncertain. Third, several studies suggest that there is not a linear change in lung function with aging, so that extrapolating from the findings in individuals in their sixth or seventh decade of life to individuals at the extremes of old age may not be warranted. Fourth, aging encompasses changes in most of the body's structures and organ systems, making it important to tease out what is a direct result of aging on the respiratory system, such as changes in lung and chest wall recoil, and what is an indirect effect of aging, such as the progressive loss of height that accompanies aging and its attendant effects on lung function. Fifth, how

The original version of the chapter has been revised. A correction to this chapter can be found at https://doi.org/10.1007/978-3-031-98371-9_9

H. L. Manning (✉)
Dartmouth-Hitchcock Medical Center, Geisel School of Medicine at Dartmouth, Hanover, NH, USA
e-mail: Harold.L.Manning@Dartmouth.edu

E. R. Swenson, A. M. Luks (eds.), *The Lungs at the Extremes of Environment and Age*, Respiratory Medicine, https://doi.org/10.1007/978-3-031-98371-9_8

representative are individuals who survive into their ninth or tenth decade of the overall population? It is plausible that part of their survival advantage entails relative resistance of their respiratory system to aging, and studies in such individuals may not reflect the effects of aging in the broader population. Finally, and perhaps most important, is the challenge of defining what constitutes "normal aging" and identifying the appropriate population to study to characterize the effect of aging on the respiratory system. Some studies have included subjects who were current or past smokers [1–3]. There is also a growing body of evidence from animal and human studies that both outdoor and indoor air pollution affect lung growth and development [4, 5] which raises the question of how much of normal aging reflects the aging process per se, and how much is related to cumulative exposure to both indoor and outdoor sources of pollution. Should studies of the effect of aging on lung function be restricted to individuals from rural areas with low levels of outdoor air pollution who also resided in homes with high indoor air quality? Or should studies of aging use individuals exposed to "average" levels of pollution? Many of these questions lack a definitive or even generally agreed-upon answer. With those caveats in mind, we'll now examine the changes in breathing that accompany aging.

Respiratory Mechanics

Changes in lung and chest wall compliance underlie many of the other changes in lung mechanics that occur with aging.

In one of the first studies to systematically examine the effects of aging, Frank and colleagues [6] studied 28 "apparently healthy" subjects who ranged in age from 50 to 89 years and found that functional residual capacity (FRC) and residual volume (RV) were higher in the elderly subjects. Although they found similar values for lung compliance in their elderly patients and in a control group of younger subjects who ranged in age from 18 to 47 years, at any given static transpulmonary pressure, lung volume was greater in the elderly patients. In other words, although the slope of the volume–pressure relationship of the lung did not differ significantly between the young and elderly subjects, there was a shift of the curve to the left in the elderly subjects. The authors reasoned that if the increase in FRC in the elderly subjects had been due to reduced elastic recoil of the lungs, transpulmonary pressure at FRC would have decreased, and if the increase in FRC were due to an increase in chest wall recoil, transpulmonary pressure at FRC would have increased. Given their finding that the increase in FRC in the elderly subjects was unaccompanied by an increase in transpulmonary pressure, they concluded that the change in FRC was due to both an increase in the elastic recoil of the chest wall and a decrease in the elastic recoil of the lungs. Pierce and Ebert [7] reported a similar increase in FRC and RV in a group of elderly patients admitted to the hospital for prostate cancer, but unlike Frank et al., they found that static lung compliance was significantly higher in the elderly patients. However, the interpretation of the Pierce study is confounded by their inclusion of subjects who had respiratory symptoms or abnormal physical findings on chest examination.

Since these initial studies, there have been a number of investigations into the effects of aging on the mechanical properties of the respiratory system, and although some studies have produced conflicting findings, some general conclusions can be drawn.

The elastic recoil of the lung decreases with age [6, 8–10], which may be related to a reduction in the number and thickness of the elastic fibers in the aging lung [11]. Men appear to lose elastic recoil faster than women [12], and loss of elastic recoil may accelerate after age 70 [13]. Although there are conflicting results about the effect of aging on static lung compliance, dynamic lung compliance decreases with aging [9, 14], presumably as a result of greater heterogeneity in the time constants among different lung regions. Lung compliance varies with lung volume in both the young and elderly, but there is less of an effect of lung volume on compliance in the elderly [15]. One potential explanation for this observation is that decreased chest wall compliance in the elderly limits expansion of the lungs and prevents them from reaching the flatter, i.e., less compliant portion of their volume–pressure relationship [15].

The chest wall can be thought of as consisting of two compartments, a rib cage compartment and a diaphragm–abdominal compartment, that together determine overall chest wall compliance, which decreases with age [15]. Estenne et al. [16] demonstrated that a decrease in both rib cage and diaphragm–abdominal compliance contributes to the decreased chest wall compliance that occurs with aging (Fig. 8.1). Decreased rib cage compliance may be related to calcification of costal cartilage and costovertebral joints and narrowing of intervertebral disk spaces; the basis for the decreased diaphragm–abdominal compliance is less clear, though increases in abdominal fat could play a role [16]. Although both the rib cage

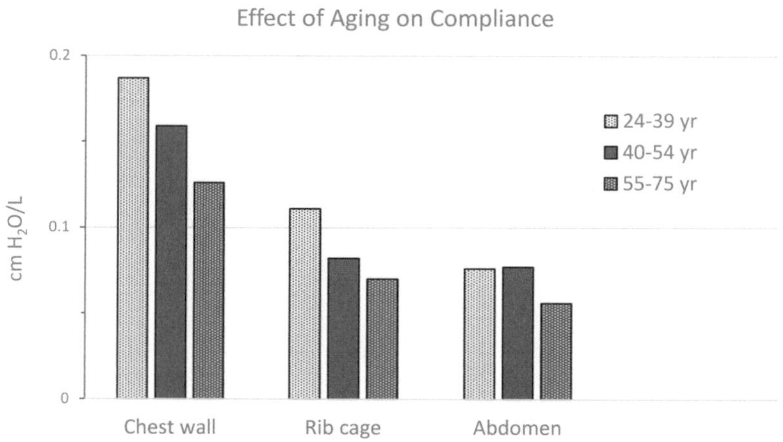

Fig. 8.1 Effect of aging on chest wall compliance and its components, rib cage and abdominal compliance. (Adapted from Estenne et al. [16])

compliance and the diaphragm–abdominal compliance decrease with aging, Rizzato and Marazzini [17] showed that in the elderly, a smaller fraction of the vital capacity displaces the rib cage and a greater fraction displaces the diaphragm–abdominal compartment. They concluded that their finding was likely a result of "changes in the joints of the thoracic skeleton." The decrease in chest wall compliance with aging exceeds any increase in lung compliance, so that total respiratory system compliance decreases with age [8].

Closing volume, the volume at which airway closure begins to occur, increases with age [9, 18, 19]. Ruff found that at a mean age of 44 years, closing volume exceeded FRC in the supine position, and by age 66, closing volume also exceeded FRC in the sitting position [19]. This finding has implications for gas exchange, which will be discussed later in this chapter. Critical closing pressure (P_{crit}), which is an expression of the tendency of the airways to collapse, increases with age [20]. The increase in P_{crit} and the accompanying increase in closing volume are a result of the loss of elastic recoil and decreased tethering of the small airways.

Expiratory flow rates at low lung volumes decrease with age [10, 21]. De Bisschop and colleagues [22] found that 86% of men and 67% of women over the age of 80 had expiratory flow limitation during tidal breathing. Frank and colleagues found that flow resistance was higher in elderly subjects [6], as did Cohn and Donoso [14] and Niewoehner and Kleinerman [23], but other studies have shown no effect of aging on airway conductance [24, 25], specific airway conductance [25, 26], or airway resistance [24].

In addition to the aforementioned changes in lung and chest wall mechanics, upper airway function is also affected by aging. Eikermann and colleagues [27] reported a number of age-related changes in upper airway function during sleep, including greater collapsibility as reflected by an increase in pharyngeal closing pressure (Fig. 8.2), and an increase in upper airway resistance. However, there was no difference in upper airway resistance between young and older subjects during wakefulness.

In summary, aging is associated with important changes in the mechanical properties of the respiratory system, including a decrease in lung elastic recoil, a decrease in rib cage and abdominal compliance, decreased expiratory flows at low lung volumes, and an increase in airway closing volume accompanied by greater collapsibility of the upper airway.

Respiratory Muscles

When skeletal muscles contract, they develop tension. In a three-dimensional structure such as the thorax, the tension developed by contracting respiratory muscles leads to pressure changes. The strength of the respiratory muscles is most often described in terms of maximal static respiratory pressures (PI_{max}, maximal inspiratory pressure, or "MIP;" and PE_{max}, maximal expiratory pressure, or "MEP"). Black and Hyatt [28] studied 120 normal subjects ranging in age from 20 to 74 years. They

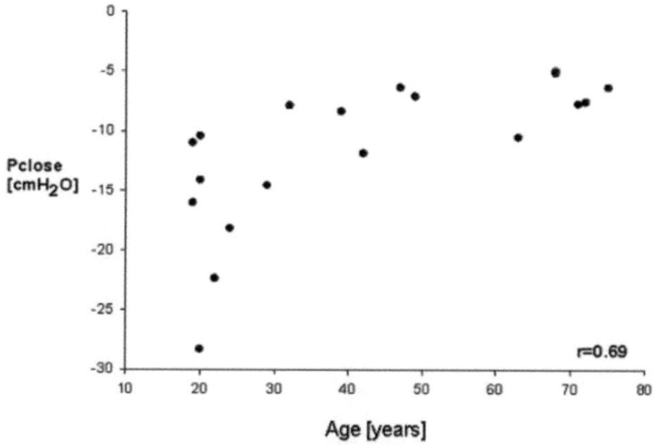

Fig. 8.2 Relationship between age and airway closing pressure (P_{close}). P_{close} refers to the decrease in airway pressure needed to cause upper airway collapse. A more negative number means that a greater pressure change is necessary to cause collapse, i.e., that the upper airway that is less collapsible. (Reprinted from Eikermann et al. [27], Copyright 2007 with permission from Elsevier)

found a "break point" of 55 years; above that, maximal respiratory pressures decreased with age, but below that, there was no correlation between age and maximal respiratory pressures. McElvaney and colleagues [29] restricted their study of maximal respiratory pressures to subjects older than 55 years of age. In contrast to Black and Hyatt, they found no relationship between age and either PI_{max} or PE_{max}, but interindividual variation was high, thereby limiting the ability to detect age-related changes without examining large numbers of subjects. In the Cardiovascular Health Study [30] in which measurements were made in more than 4000 subjects aged 65 years and older, there was a progressive decline in maximal respiratory pressures with aging; the age-related decline was more pronounced in men than women (Fig. 8.3).

Maximal respiratory pressures reflect the combined output of the many respiratory muscles; transdiaphragmatic pressure, P_{di}, reflects the strength of the diaphragm. Tolep et al. [31] compared P_{di} in nine young subjects, mean age 24 years, with that of ten elderly subjects, mean age 68 years, and found that over a range of lung volumes, mean P_{di} was significantly lower in the elderly subjects, though as was the case with maximal respiratory pressures, there was substantial variability among subjects within each group (Fig. 8.4). Polkey and colleagues [32] studied a slightly larger group of subjects and measured P_{di} generated during a maximal sniff effort and bilateral cervical magnetic stimulation of the phrenic nerve roots. They found that although mean values for P_{di} were significantly lower in the elderly for both sniff efforts and magnetic stimulation, the differences were relatively small, with considerable overlap between groups.

In addition to measures of respiratory muscle strength, one might consider the efficiency of the respiratory muscles, as reflected in their oxygen consumption relative to ventilation. In a group of 37 normal male subjects ranging in age from 23 to

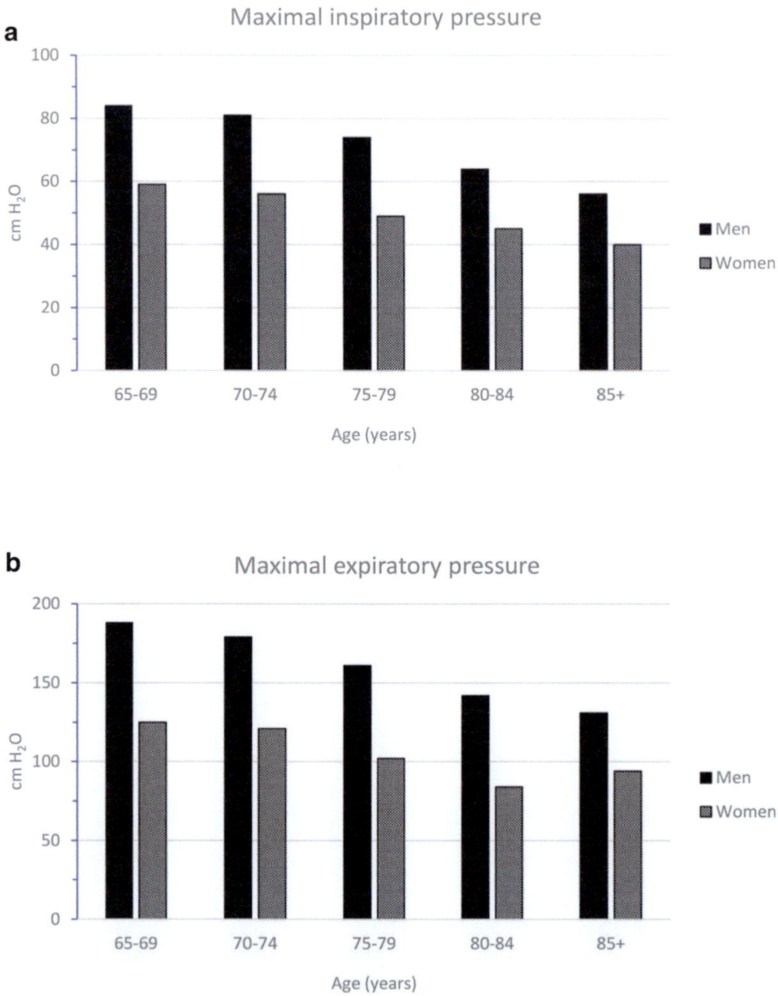

Fig. 8.3 Effect of aging on maximal inspiratory pressure (**a**) and maximal expiratory pressure (**b**). Although not shown in the figure, the number of subjects in the 85+ group was much smaller than the other age groups. (Adapted from the data of Enright et al. [30])

77 years, Takishima et al. [33] stimulated an increase in ventilation by increasing dead space in their subjects and found that $\log \dot{V}O_{2resp} / \dot{V}_E$ increased with age, which they suggested could be due to age-related increases in airway resistance or decreases in chest wall compliance and respiratory muscle strength.

In summary, the combined strength of the respiratory muscles and the strength of the diaphragm in particular all decrease significantly with age, though the change is not marked, and to some degree, the age-related changes are overshadowed by large interindividual variation among individuals of similar age. As we age, the

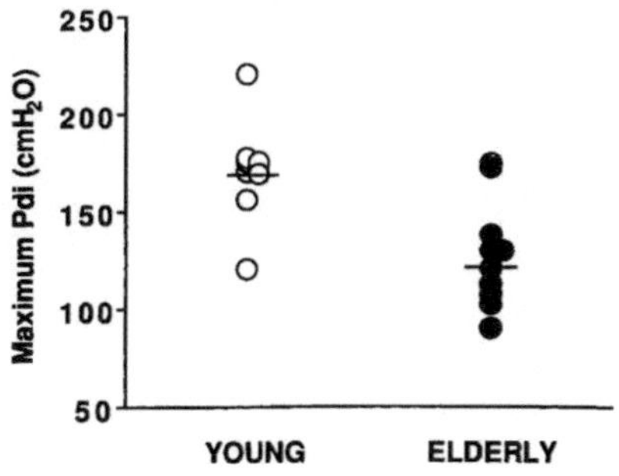

Fig. 8.4 Maximal transdiaphragmatic pressure (Pdi) in young and elderly subjects. (Reprinted with permission of the American Thoracic Society. Copyright © 2024 American Thoracic Society. All rights reserved. Tolep et al. [31])

respiratory muscles become less efficient in that at any given level of ventilation, the respiratory muscles consume greater quantities of oxygen.

Pulmonary Function Testing

Studies of the effect of aging on lung function fall into two general categories. *Cross-sectional* studies examine lung function at a single point in time in individuals spanning a range of ages to determine whether there is a significant correlation between age and the measure of lung function of interest. In contrast, *longitudinal* studies involve measurements that are repeated in the same individuals at different points in time. The two types of studies have generally shown similar relationships between aging and measures of lung function, though estimates of the magnitude of the effect often differ.

Lung Volumes

Total lung capacity (TLC), the maximum volume to which the respiratory system can be inflated, represents the balance point between the maximum force that can be generated by the inspiratory muscles and the elastic recoil of the lung and chest wall. The changes in the mechanical properties of the lung and chest wall have offsetting effects on total lung capacity (TLC). The decrease in lung elastic recoil that occurs with aging would tend to increase TLC, whereas the increase in chest wall elastic recoil would tend to decrease it. If one accounts for the decrease in height that occurs with aging, the net result is that there is no significant effect of aging on TLC [34, 35].

FRC represents the balance point between the inward (positive) elastic recoil of the lung and the negative (outward) elastic recoil of the chest wall. In this case, the changes in lung and chest wall mechanics both act in the same direction, and most studies show that FRC increases significantly with aging [7, 14].

In the young, residual volume (RV) is determined by a balance of forces, i.e., the negative or outward elastic recoil of the chest wall versus the strength of the expiratory muscles (aided by a small contribution from the elastic recoil of the lung). However, as we age, airway closure becomes the key determinant of residual volume. A consistent finding among studies is that RV increases with age [7, 14, 15, 35], as does RV/TLC [8, 21, 34], a consequence of the decreased lung elastic recoil and the accompanying tendency for airway collapse at higher lung volumes that occurs with aging.

Given the lack of change in TLC but a progressive increase in RV, vital capacity predictably decreases with age [36].

Spirometry

A consistent finding is that the forced expiratory volume in one second (FEV_1), the forced vital capacity (FVC), and the FEV_1/FVC ratio all decrease with age [21, 36, 37]. Burrows et al. [38] showed that the decline in FEV_1 begins around age 35, and the rate of fall increases with age [38, 39] (Fig. 8.5).

Diffusing Capacity

Donevan et al. [40] measured the diffusing capacity in 24 normal subjects who ranged in age from 20 to 50 years, and found that the diffusing capacity at rest and with exercise decreased with increasing age, which they speculated might be due to an accompanying decrease in cardiac output with increasing age. The finding of an age-related decline in diffusing capacity has been confirmed repeatedly [41–44] (Fig. 8.6), though interindividual variation is high. Hamer [41] found that the membrane component of the diffusing capacity decreased with age, but pulmonary capillary blood volume did not. In contrast, Georges [42] reported that both components of the diffusing capacity, i.e., the membrane component and pulmonary capillary blood volume, both decreased with age, though not in a linear fashion. Aging is associated with dilation of the airspaces [45], a process often referred to as "senile emphysema," which may contribute to the decrease in diffusing capacity in the elderly [43].

In summary, FEV_1, FVC, FEV_1/FVC, and the diffusing capacity all decrease with age, whereas RV and likely FRC increase with age. TLC is largely unaffected by aging during adulthood.

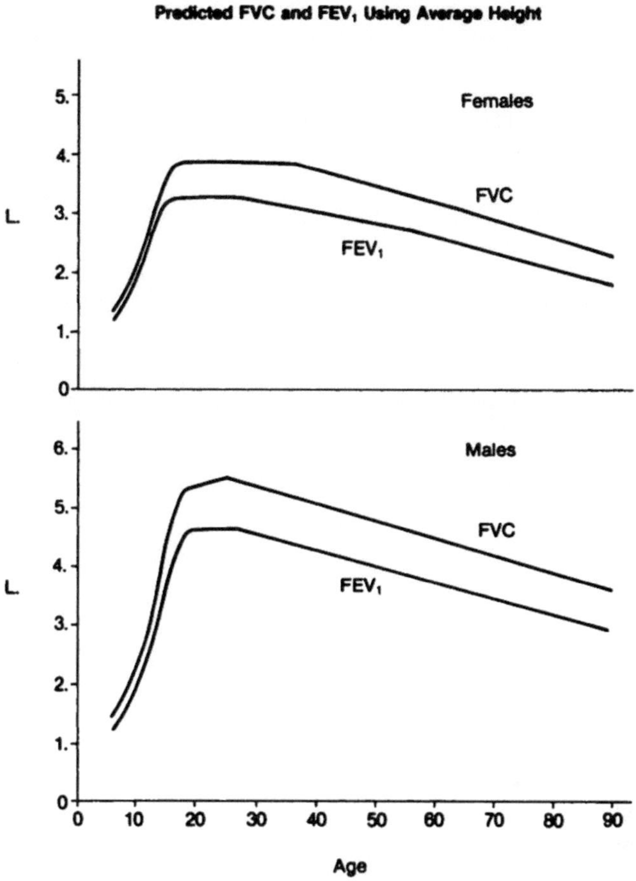

Fig. 8.5 Change in FEV_1 and FVC with age. (Reprinted from Burrows et al. [72], Copyright 1983 with permission from Elsevier)

Gas Exchange

Aging has effects on both oxygenation and CO_2 elimination, which are ultimately related to the accompanying age-related changes in lung mechanics.

Healthy elderly individuals have a lower partial pressure of oxygen (PO_2) [46, 47] than normal young subjects. Estimates of the age-related decline in arterial PO_2 range from approximately 0.11–0.43 mmHg/year [46–48]. The decrease in arterial PO_2 is accompanied by an increase in the alveolar–arterial oxygen difference ($[A\text{-}a]\Delta O_2$) [2, 47, 48]. Kanber et al. [2] reported a mean $[A\text{-}a]\Delta O_2$ of 7 mmHg in a group of young subjects whose average age was 34, and a mean $[A\text{-}a]\Delta O_2$ of 14 mmHg in a group of elderly subjects whose mean age was 72 years. Of note, most of the subjects in the study were current or past smokers. Mellemgaard [48] reported that the $[A\text{-}a]\Delta O_2$ increased by approximately 0.2 mmHg/year. However,

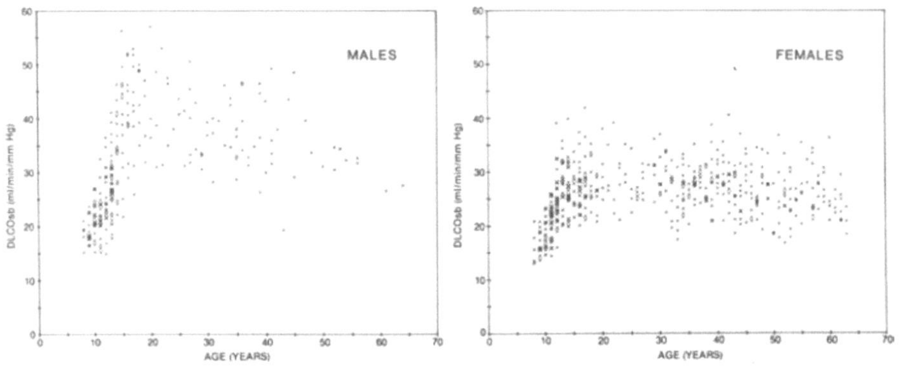

Fig. 8.6 Change in DL_{CO} with age. Values decrease starting at approximately age 20. (Reprinted with permission of the American Thoracic Society. Copyright © 2024 American Thoracic Society. All rights reserved. Paoletti et al. [43])

the changes in PO_2 and $[A\text{-}a]\Delta O_2$ may not progress beyond a certain age. Guenard and Marthan [3] studied 74 healthy subjects who ranged in age from 69 to 104 years [3]. They found no correlation between age and either arterial PO_2 or $[A\text{-}a]\Delta O_2$, but at most ages, there was significant interindividual variation, making it difficult to know whether their results reflect a true plateau in age-related changes in oxygenation or simply too few subjects to detect in a change in the setting of marked interindividual variation.

Fowler [49] measured dead space in ten young subjects whose mean age was 28 years and in 11 subjects whose mean age was 60 years; none of the subjects had "clinical or fluoroscopic evidence of cardio-respiratory disease." He found that there was a small, but not statistically significant, increase in dead space in the older subjects; that was true whether dead space was measured as an absolute volume or as a fraction of tidal volume. In contrast, Tenney and Miller [50] measured dead space ventilation in 18 elderly, normal men between the ages of 68 and 89. Based on a high minute ventilation but normal values for alveolar and arterial partial pressure of carbon dioxide (PCO_2), they concluded that dead space ventilation must represent a disproportionately large fraction of total ventilation. Mellemgaard [48] also found an increase in physiological dead space with increasing age.

Studies of the effect of age on the distribution of ventilation offer insight into the mechanisms underlying the changes in gas exchange that occur with aging. Holland et al. [1] used radioactive xenon to measure the distribution of ventilation in six individuals who ranged in age from 65 to 75 years and compared them to previous findings in a group of young subjects whose age averaged 35 years. In the elderly subjects, ventilation during tidal breathing was not preferentially distributed to the lower lung zones, as it was in the younger subjects, which they attributed to the significantly higher closing volumes in the older subjects, five out of six of whom had closing capacities that exceeded FRC. Other studies have confirmed that the distribution of ventilation is less uniform in the elderly [51], who also have greater ventilation–perfusion inequality [47] (Fig. 8.7).

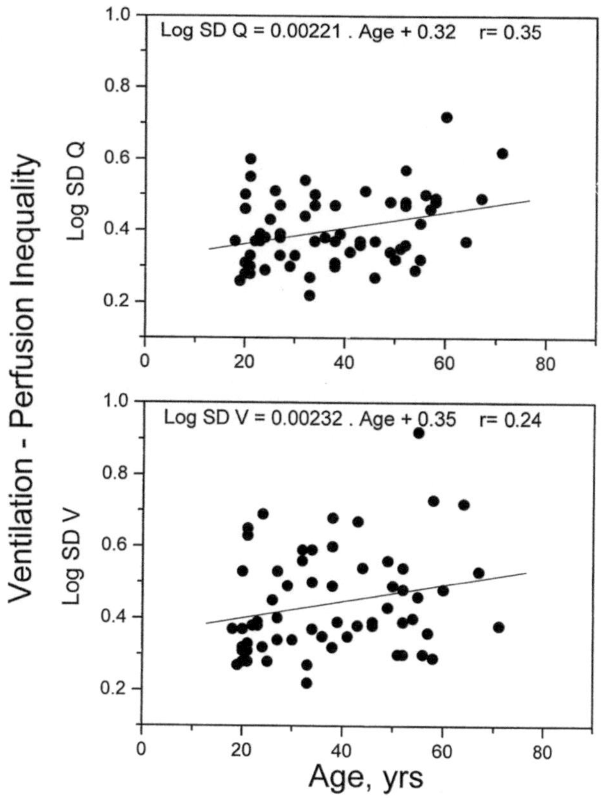

Fig. 8.7 Effect of aging on ventilation–perfusion (V/Q) inequality. Log SD Q and Log SD V are measures of the regional dispersion in pulmonary blood and ventilation, respectively. Aging is accompanied by a significant increase in V/Q inequality. (Reprinted with permission of the American Thoracic Society. Copyright © 2024 American Thoracic Society. All rights reserved. Cardus et al. [47])

Control of Breathing

The respiratory control system can be described in terms of the ventilatory response to chemical stimuli such as hypoxia and hypercapnia, and the response to an added load. However, the ventilatory response reflects not only the sensitivity of the respiratory control system to stimuli but also the mechanical properties of the respiratory system, which may modify the output of the respiratory system, i.e., ventilation. The pressure measured during the first 0.1 s of an occluded breath, $P_{0.1}$, may more closely reflect respiratory drive, particularly when mechanical abnormalities are present [52], and the $P_{0.1}$ response has been used to characterize the sensitivity to respiratory stimuli. There are conflicting data about the effect of aging on the ventilatory response to chemical stimuli. In a cross-sectional study of 63 subjects, Patrick and Howard [53] reported that in older subjects, the tidal volume response to CO_2 was only 69% of that of the younger subjects, but there was no significant difference when the response to hypercapnia was expressed in terms of total ventilation. However, it is worth noting that in their study, there were only nine "older" subjects, and the older subjects had a mean age of only 44 years. Kronenberg and Drage [54] (1973) and Peterson et al. [55] both found that compared to young subjects, the ventilatory responses to both hypoxemia and hypercapnia were reduced by approximately 50% in healthy elderly subjects. In the Peterson study, the decreased ventilatory responses were characterized by smaller tidal volumes and lower flow rates and by proportional reductions in the $P_{0.1}$ response; there were no significant differences in measures of respiratory timing. Since the older subjects demonstrated only minor changes in pulmonary mechanics, these investigators concluded that the older subjects had a reduction in respiratory motor output, i.e., decreased respiratory drive, as the basis for the decreased ventilatory responses. Garcia-Rio et al. [56] confirmed the finding of a decreased $P_{0.1}$ response to hypercapnia and hypoxemia in the elderly. In contrast to the aforementioned findings, Ahmed and colleagues [57] assessed the ventilatory response to 25 min of hypoxemia and found no difference between the young subjects (mean age 29) and the older subjects (mean age 62).

Rubin et al. [58] compared the response to CO_2 with and without an inspiratory resistive load in 18 young subjects with a mean age of 25 years with the response in ten older subjects who had a mean age of 66 years. There was a trend toward higher ventilatory and $P_{0.1}$ responses to hypercapnia in the young subjects that did not achieve statistical significance, but failure to achieve significance may have been due to the small number of subjects combined with marked interindividual variation within each of the groups. In the presence of an inspiratory resistive load, both the young and elderly subjects had an increase in the $P_{0.1}$ response and a decreased ventilatory response compared to the unloaded condition, but there was no significant difference between the groups. Thus, in this study, young and elderly subjects responded similarly to chemical stimuli as well as a mechanical load.

There is still uncertainty about the mechanism(s) governing the ventilatory response to exercise. Although the chemoreceptors may play a role in normal individuals, evidence suggests that ventilation may increase normally during exercise, even in the absence of central chemoreceptor function [59]. Brischetto and colleagues [60] compared the ventilatory responses to CO_2 and exercise in ten young and ten older patients and found that although the mean ventilatory response to CO_2 was reduced in the elderly subjects, the older subjects had an increased ventilatory response to exercise. This was true whether ventilation was related to CO_2 production, O_2 uptake, or work rate, which they speculated was necessary to offset the increased dead space ventilation that accompanies aging. The finding of an increased ventilatory response to exercise was confirmed by Poulin et al. [61], who found a linear relationship between ventilation and CO_2 production in both men and women (Fig. 8.8).

In addition to changes in chemosensitivity, perception of vagal stimuli may be affected by aging. Newnham and Hamilton [62] induced cough with distilled water in 20 elderly subjects with a mean age of 83 years and 20 young subjects with a mean age of 27 years, and found a significant decrease in cough frequency in the elderly subjects (Fig. 8.9). It is unclear whether the decreased sensitivity of the cough reflex in the elderly reflects changes in vagal receptor function or changes in the central processing of vagal receptor inputs.

In summary, the bulk of evidence indicates that the ventilatory response to chemical stimuli decreases with age; there may also be decreased responsiveness to vagal

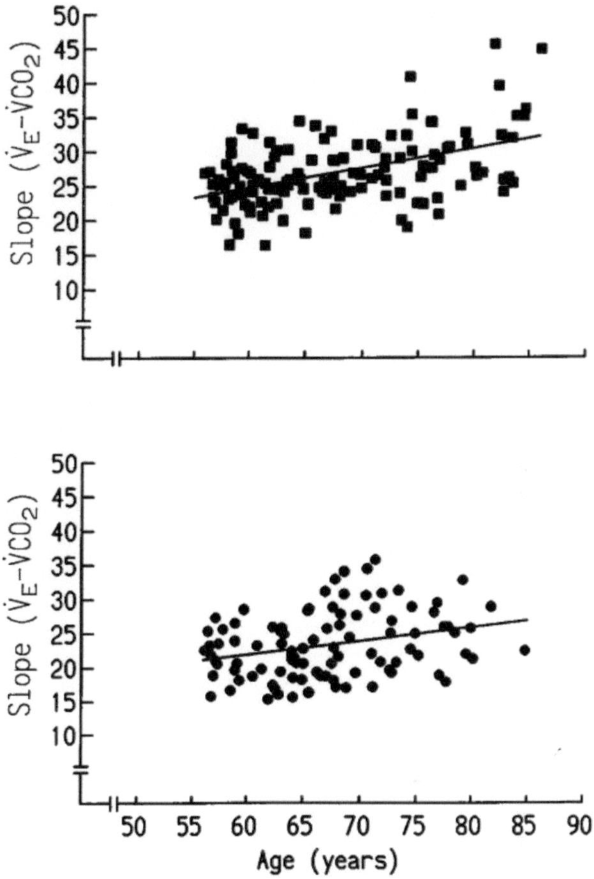

Fig. 8.8 Effect of aging on the ventilatory response to exercise. In both men (top panel) and women (bottom panel), the ventilatory response to exercise, expressed as the slope of the relationship between ventilation ($\dot{V}_E$) and CO_2 production ($\dot{V}_{CO_2}$), increases with aging. (Reprinted with permission of the American Thoracic Society. Copyright © 2024 American Thoracic Society. All rights reserved. Poulin et al. [61])

stimuli. Whether these changes are a result of altered receptor function or altered central processing of the sensory inputs is unclear. In contrast to the decreased ventilatory response to chemical stimuli, the ventilatory response to exercise is increased in the elderly.

Respiratory Sensation

Psychophysics is the study of the relationship between physical stimuli and the sensations they elicit. A detailed discussion of psychophysics is beyond the scope of this chapter, but some basic principles of psychophysics are helpful in understanding how respiratory stimuli are perceived. Respiratory sensations can be characterized by their threshold, i.e., the minimum stimulus intensity that can be detected, and/or by describing the relationship between the magnitude of a sensory stimulus and the resulting intensity of the perception. Much of the foundational work in the

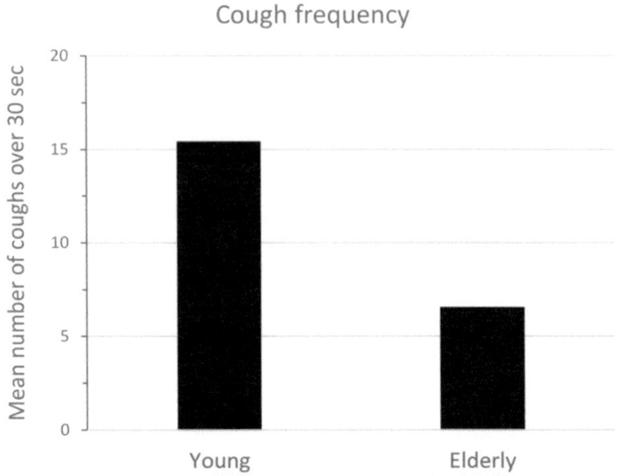

Fig. 8.9 Cough sensitivity in young and elderly subjects. In response to nebulized distilled water, young subjects had significantly greater mean cough frequency over a 30-s interval than elderly subjects. (Adapted from Newnham and Hamilton [62])

field of psychophysics was undertaken by Stevens [63, 64], who showed that the relationship between the magnitude of a stimulus and the intensity of the resulting sensation could be described by a power function: $\Psi = k\, I^n$, where Ψ is the sensory judgment of the stimulus, k is a scaling constant, I is the physical magnitude of the stimulus, and the exponent n is the relative sensitivity. The exponent n can be used to describe the sensitivity of individuals to various stimuli, including respiratory stimuli.

Tack and colleagues compared the sensitivity of young and elderly subjects to elastic [65] and resistive [66] loads and found that the Stevens' exponent was greater for young than elderly subjects for both types of loads. Altose [67] confirmed the findings of a smaller exponent for resistive loads in the elderly and showed that the difference between young and elderly subjects persisted when airway pressure (rather than the magnitude of the resistance) was used as the physical stimulus underlying the sensation.

Another way of characterizing the sensitivity to mechanical stimuli is by the threshold for detection of an added load. Allen et al. [68] compared the threshold for detecting resistive loads during normal tidal breathing and found that the threshold for both inspiratory and expiratory resistive loads was significantly higher in the group of individuals aged 65 or older than in the group who ranged in age from 20 to 39 years (Fig. 8.10).

Murtolahti [69] modified nasal resistance, and found that, similar to added external resistive loads, the threshold for detecting an increase in nasal resistance was significantly higher in the older subjects, though both young and elderly subjects responded to the increase in nasal resistance by decreasing their flow rates.

Although the stimulus (or stimuli) for breathlessness during exercise is uncertain, at a standard $\dot{V}O_2$ Ofir et al. [70] found that older individuals had higher breathlessness ratings than younger individuals, and the slope of breathlessness rating/$\dot{V}O_2$ was steeper in the older subjects. The study did not report the slope of leg discomfort ratings/$\dot{V}O_2$, so it is impossible to know whether the higher

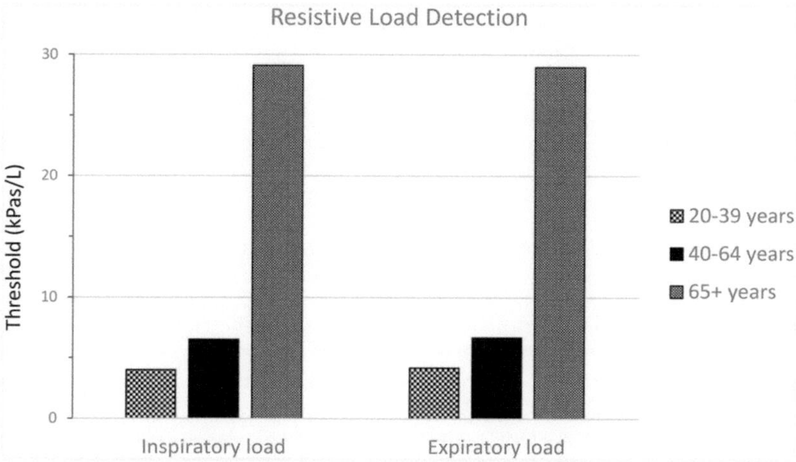

Fig. 8.10 The threshold for both inspiratory and expiratory resistive load detection was significantly higher in elderly subjects than in young subjects. (Adapted from Allen et al. [68])

breathlessness ratings in the elderly reflected a specific effect on the processing of respiratory-related information or a nonspecific effect of aging on the rating of aversive stimuli in general. In contrast to the findings of Ofri et al., Faisal et al. [71] induced breathlessness by adding dead space to the breathing circuit during exercise and found breathlessness ratings increased to a similar extent in both the young and elderly subjects.

In summary, whether sensitivity is expressed as the Stevens exponent or the threshold for load detection, healthy elderly individuals are less sensitive than young individuals to both elastic or resistive loads. Since most respiratory diseases are associated with increased elastic or resistive loads, one might hypothesize that elderly patients are more likely to develop and present with symptoms later in the course of their illness.

Conclusion

Aging is associated with diverse and important changes in the physiology of the respiratory system, though the extent to which the changes reflect aging alone versus cumulative exposure to a variety of environmental insults is unknown. These age-related changes lead to measurable effects on gas exchange and common clinical tests of lung function, affect how older individuals perceive and respond to a variety of respiratory stimuli, and could account for some of the differences in how young and older individuals present with respiratory disease.

References

1. Holland J, Milic-Emili J, Macklem PT, Bates DV. Regional distribution of pulmonary ventilation and perfusion in elderly subjects. J Clin Invest. 1968;47(1):81–92.
2. Kanber GJ, King FW, Eshchar YR, Sharp JT. The alveolar-arterial oxygen gradient in young and elderly men during air and oxygen breathing. Am Rev Respir Dis. 1968;97(3):376–81.
3. Guénard H, Marthan R. Pulmonary gas exchange in elderly subjects. Eur Respir J. 1996;9(12):2573–7.
4. Gauderman WJ, Avol E, Gilliland F, Vora H, Thomas D, Berhane K, et al. The effect of air pollution on lung development from 10 to 18 years of age. N Engl J Med. 2004;351(11):1057–67.
5. Mauad T, Rivero DHRF, De Oliveira RC, Lichtenfels AJDFC, Guimarães ET, De Andre PA, et al. Chronic exposure to ambient levels of urban particles affects mouse lung development. Am J Respir Crit Care Med. 2008;178:721–8.
6. Frank NR, Mead J, Ferris BG. The mechanical behavior of the lungs in healthy elderly persons. J Clin Invest. 1957;36(12):1680–7.
7. Pierce JA, Ebert RV. The elastic properties of the lungs in the aged. J Lab Clin Med. 1958;51(1):63.
8. Turner JM, Mead J, Wohl ME. Elasticity of human lungs in relation to age. J Appl Physiol. 1968;25:664–71.
9. Begin R, Renzetti AD, Bigler AH, Watanabe S. Flow and age dependence of airway closure and dynamic compliance. J Appl Physiol. 1975;38:199–207.
10. Knudson RJ, Clark DF, Kennedy TC, Knudson DE. Effect of aging alone on mechanical properties of the normal adult human lung. J Appl Physiol. 1977;43:1054–62.
11. Wright RR. Elastic tissue of normal and emphysematous lungs. A tridimensional histologic study. Am J Pathol. 1961;39:355–67.
12. Bode FR, Dosman J, Martin RR, Ghezzo H, Macklem PT. Age and sex differences in lung elasticity, and in closing capacity in nonsmokers. J Appl Physiol. 1976;41:129–35.
13. Knudson RJ, Lebowitz MD, Holberg CJ, Burrows B. Changes in the normal maximal expiratory flow-volume curve with growth and aging. Am Rev Respir Dis. 1983;127(6):725–34.
14. Cohn JE, Donoso HD. Mechanical properties of lung in normal men over 60 years old. J Clin Invest. 1963;42:1406–10.
15. Mittman C, Edelman NH, Norris AH, Shock NW. Relationship between chest wall and pulmonary compliance and age. J Appl Physiol. 1965;20:1211–6.
16. Estenne M, Yernault JC, De Troyer A. Rib cage and diaphragm-abdomen compliance in humans: effects of age and posture. J Appl Physiol. 1985;59:1842–8.
17. Rizzato G, Marazzini L. Thoracoabdominal mechanics in elderly men. J Appl Physiol. 1970;28(4):457–60.
18. Anthonisen NR, Danson J, Robertson PC, Ross WRD. Airway closure as a function of age. Respir Physiol. 1969;8:58–65.
19. Ruff F. Effects of age and posture on closing volume. Scand. J Respir Dis. 1974;55(sup.85):190–200.
20. Gelb AF, Zamel N. Effect of aging on lung mechanics in healthy nonsmokers. Chest. 1975;68:538–41.
21. Gibson GJ, Pride NB, O'cain C, Quagliato R. Sex and age differences in pulmonary mechanics in normal nonsmoking subjects. J Appl Physiol. 1976;41:20–5.
22. de Bisschop C, Marty ML, Tessier JF, Barberger-Gateau P, Dartigues JF, Guénard H. Expiratory flow limitation and obstruction in the elderly. Eur Respir J. 2005;26:594–601.
23. Niewoehner DE, Kleinerman J. Morphologic basis of pulmonary resistance in the human lung and effects of aging. J Appl Physiol. 1974;36(4):412–8.
24. Briscoe WA, Dubois AB. The relationship between airway resistance, airway conductance and lung volume in subjects of different age and body size. J Clin Invest. 1958;37:1279–85.
25. Pelzer AM, Thomson ML. Effect of age, sex, stature, and smoking habits on human airway conductance. J Appl Physiol. 1966;21(2):469–76.

26. Berry RB, Pai UP, Fairshter RD. Effect of age on changes in flow rates and airway conductance after a deep breath. J Appl Physiol. 1990;68(2):635–43.
27. Eikermann M, Jordan AS, Chamberlin NL, Gautam S, Wellman A, Lo YL, et al. The influence of aging on pharyngeal collapsibility during sleep. Chest. 2007;131:1702–9.
28. Black LF, Hyatt RE. Maximal respiratory pressures: normal values and relationship to age and sex. Am Rev Respir Dis. 1969;99:696–702.
29. McElvaney G, Blackie S, Morrison NJ, Wilcox PG, Fairbarn MS, Pardy RL. Maximal static respiratory pressures in the normal elderly. Am Rev Respir Dis. 1989;139:277–81.
30. Enright PL, Kronmal RA, Manolio TA, Schenker MB, Hyatt RE. Respiratory muscle strength in the elderly: correlates and reference values. Am J Respir Crit Care Med. 1994;149:430–8.
31. Tolep K, Higgins N, Muza S, Criner G, Kelsen SG. Comparison of diaphragm strength between healthy adult elderly and young men. Am J Respir Crit Care Med. 1995;152(2):677–82.
32. Polkey MI, Lou HM, Hughes PD, Hamnegård CH, Lyons D, Green M, et al. The contractile properties of the elderly human diaphragm. Am J Respir Crit Care Med. 1997;155:1560–4.
33. Takishima T, Shindoh C, Kikuchi Y, Hida W, Inoue H. Aging effect on oxygen consumption of respiratory muscles in humans. J Appl Physiol. 1990;69:14–20.
34. Boren HG, Kory RC, Syner JC. The veterans administration-army cooperative study of pulmonary function. II. The lung volume and its subdivisions in normal men. Am J Med. 1966;41:96–114.
35. McClaran SR, Babcock MA, Pegelow DF, Reddan WG, Dempsey JA. Longitudinal effects of aging on lung function at rest and exercise in healthy active fit elderly adults. J Appl Physiol. 1995;78:1957–68.
36. Ashley F, Kannel WB, Sorlie PD, Masson R. Pulmonary function: relation to aging, cigarette habit, and mortality: the Framingham study. Ann Intern Med. 1975;82:739–45.
37. Morris JF, Temple WP, Koski A. Normal values for the ratio of one second forced expiratory volume to forced vital capacity. Am Rev Respir Dis. 1973;108:1000–3.
38. Burrows B, Lebowitz MD, Camilli AE, Knudson RJ. Longitudinal changes in forced expiratory volume in one second in adults. Methodologic considerations and findings in healthy nonsmokers. Am Rev Respir Dis. 1986;133:974–80.
39. Ware JH, Dockery DW, Louis TA, Xu X, Ferris BG, Speizer FE. Longitudinal and cross-sectional estimates of pulmonary function decline in never-smoking adults. Am J Epidemiol. 1990;132:685–700.
40. Donevan RE, Palmer WH, Varvis CJ, Bates DV. Influence of age on pulmonary diffusing capacity. J Appl Physiol. 1959;14:483–92.
41. Hamer NA. The effect of age on the components of the pulmonary diffusing capacity. Clin Sci. 1962;23:85–93.
42. Georges R, Saumon G, Loiseau A. The relationship of age to pulmonary membrane conductance and capillary blood volume. Am Rev Respir Dis. 1978;117:1069–78.
43. Paoletti P, Viegi G, Pistelli G, Di Pede F, Fazzi P, Polato R, et al. Reference equations for the single-breath diffusing capacity. A cross-sectional analysis and effect of body size and age. Am Rev Respir Dis. 1985;132:806–13.
44. Ren WY, Li L, Zhao RY, Zhu L. Age-associated changes in pulmonary function: a comparison of pulmonary function parameters in healthy young adults and the elderly living in Shanghai. Chin Med J. 2012;125:3064–8.
45. Thurlbeck W. The internal surface area of nonemphysematous lungs. Am Rev Respir Dis. 1967;95:765–73.
46. Sorbini CA, Grassi V, Solinas E, Muiesan G. Arterial oxygen tension in relation to age in healthy subjects. Respiration. 1968;25:3–13.
47. Cardús J, Burgos F, Diaz O, Roca J, Barberà JA, Marrades RM, et al. Increase in pulmonary ventilation-perfusion inequality with age in healthy individuals. Am J Respir Crit Care Med. 1997;156:648–53.
48. Mellemgaard K. The alveolar-arterial oxygen difference: its size and components in normal man. Acta Physiol Scand. 1966;67:10–20.

49. Fowler WS. Lung function studies. V. Respiratory dead space in old age and in pulmonary emphysema. J Clin Invest. 1950;29:1439–44.
50. Tenney SM, Miller RM. Dead space ventilation in old age. J Appl Physiol. 1956;9:321–7.
51. Edelman NH, Mittman C, Norris AH, Shock NW. Effects of respiratory pattern on age differences in ventilation uniformity. J Appl Physiol. 1968;24:49–53.
52. Whitelaw WA, Derenne JP, Milic-Emili J. Occlusion pressure as a measure of respiratory center output cm conscious man. Respir Physiol. 1975;23:181–99.
53. Patrick JM, Howard A. The influence of age, sex, body size and lung size on the control and pattern of breathing during CO_2 inhalation in Caucasians. Respir Physiol. 1972;16:337–50.
54. Kronenberg RS, Drage CW. Attenuation of the ventilatory and heart rate responses to hypoxia and hypercapnia with aging in normal men. J Clin Invest. 1973;52:1812–9.
55. Peterson DD, Pack AI, Silage DA, Fishman AP. Effects of aging on ventilatory and occlusion pressure responses to hypoxia and hypercapnia. Am Rev Respir Dis. 1981;124:387–91.
56. García-Río F, Villamor A, Gómez-Mendieta A, Lores V, Rojo B, Ramírez T, et al. The progressive effects of ageing on chemosensitivity in healthy subjects. Respir Med. 2007;101:2192–8.
57. Ahmed M, Giesbrecht GG, Serrette C, Georgopoulos D, Anthonisen NR. Ventilatory response to hypoxia in elderly humans. Respir Physiol. 1991;83:343–51.
58. Rubin S, Tack M, Cherniack NS. Effect of aging on respiratory responses to CO_2 and inspiratory resistive loads. J Gerontol. 1982;37:306–12.
59. Manning HL, Leiter JC. Respiratory control and respiratory sensation in a patient with a ganglioglioma within the dorsocaudal brain stem. Am J Respir Crit Care Med. 2000;161:2100–6.
60. Brischetto MJ, Millman RP, Peterson DD. Effects of aging on ventilatory response to exercise and CO_2. J Appl Physiol. 1984;56:1143–50.
61. Poulin MJ, Cunningham DA, Paterson DH, Rechnitzer PA, Ecclestone NA, Koval JJ. Ventilatory response to exercise in men and women 55 to 86 years of age. Am J Respir Crit Care Med. 1994;149:408–15.
62. Newnham DM, Hamilton SJC. Sensitivity of the cough reflex in young and elderly subjects. Age Ageing. 1997;26:185–8.
63. Stevens SS. Neural events and the psychophysical law. Science. 1970;170:1043–50.
64. Stevens SS. On the psychophysical law. Psychol Rev. 1957;64:153–81.
65. Tack M, Altose MD, Cherniack NS. Effect of aging on respiratory sensations produced by elastic loads. J Appl Physiol. 1981;50:844–50.
66. Tack M, Altose MD, Cherniack NS. Effect of aging on the perception of resistive ventilatory loads. Am Rev Respir Dis. 1982;126:463–7.
67. Altose MD, Leitner J, Cherniack NS. Effects of age and respiratory efforts on the perception of resistive ventilatory loads. J Gerontol. 1985;40:147–53.
68. Allen SC, Vassallo M, Khattab A. The threshold for sensing airflow resistance during tidal breathing rises in old age: implications for elderly patients with obstructive airways diseases. Age Ageing. 2009;38:548–52.
69. Murtolahti S, Crouse UK, Pahkala R, Warren DW, Laine-Alava MT. Perception and respiratory responses of the upper airway mechanism to added resistance with aging. Laryngoscope Investig Otolaryngol. 2017;2:417–22.
70. Ofir D, Laveneziana P, Webb KA, Lam YM, O'Donnell DE. Sex differences in the perceived intensity of breathlessness during exercise with advancing age. J Appl Physiol. 2008;104:1583–93.
71. Faisal A, Webb KA, Guenette JA, Jensen D, Neder JA, O'Donnell DE. Effect of age-related ventilatory inefficiency on respiratory sensation during exercise. Respir Physiol Neurobiol. 2015;205:129–39.
72. Burrows B, et al. A descriptive analysis of the growth and decline of the FVC and FEV1. Chest. 1983;83:717–24.

Correction to: The Lungs at the Extremes of Environment and Age

Erik R. Swenson and Andrew M. Luks

Correction to:
E. R. Swenson, A. M. Luks (eds.), ***The Lungs at the Extremes of Environment and Age,*** **Respiratory Medicine, https://doi.org/10.1007/978-3-031-98371-9**

This book was recently published, but the metadata of the following chapters are misplaced in the final print version:

Chapter 6: Comparative Lung Physiology at Environmental Extremes
Chapter 8: The Elderly Lung and Breathing

The updated version of these chapters can be found at
https://doi.org/10.1007/978-3-031-98371-9_6
https://doi.org/10.1007/978-3-031-98371-9_8

E. R. Swenson, A. M. Luks (eds.), *The Lungs at the Extremes of Environment and Age*, Respiratory Medicine, https://doi.org/10.1007/978-3-031-98371-9_9

Index

E. R. Swenson, A. M. Luks (eds.), *The Lungs at the Extremes of Environment and Age*, Respiratory Medicine, https://doi.org/10.1007/978-3-031-98371-9

MIX
Papier aus verantwortungsvollen Quellen
Paper from responsible sources
FSC® C105338

If you have any concerns about our products,
you can contact us on
ProductSafety@springernature.com

In case Publisher is established outside the EU,
the EU authorized representative is:
Springer Nature Customer Service Center GmbH
Europaplatz 3, 69115 Heidelberg, Germany

Printed by Libri Plureos GmbH
in Hamburg, Germany